# Let Your Body

*We are not human beings, who have spiritual experiences,*
*But spiritual beings that have human experiences.*

*WILLIGIS JÄGER,* Die Welle ist das Meer – Mystische Spiritualität

# Let Your Body Speak

## The Essential Nature of Our Organs

**Ewald Kliegel**

**Illustrations by Anne Heng**

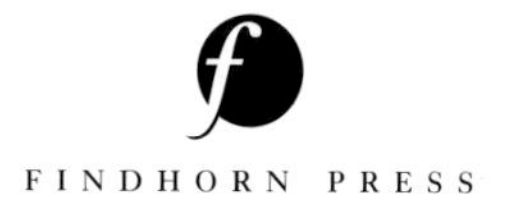

FINDHORN PRESS

English edition published by Findhorn Press, Scotland, 2013

Originally published in German

Original title: *Organwesen*



ISBN 978-1-84409-626-8



A CIP record for this title is available from the British Library.

Cover and inside illustrations by Anne Heng

Translation by Sabine Weeke

Edited by Jacqui Lewis
Cover design by Dragon Design, UK, and Thierry Bogliolo
Text designed in Kingfisher by Geoff Green Book Design, Cambridge, CB24 4RA
Printed and bound in the EU

Published by
Findhorn Press
117–121 High Street,
Forres IV36 1AB,
Scotland, UK

*t* +44 (0)1309 690582
*f* +44 (0)131 777 2711

*e* info@findhornpress.com
www.findhornpress.com

**Disclaimer**
The information in this book is given in good faith and is neither intended to diagnose any physical or mental condition nor to serve as a substitute for informed medical advice or care.
Please contact your health professional for medical advice and treatment. Neither author nor publisher can be held liable by any person for any loss or damage whatsoever which may arise from the use of this book or any of the information therein.

# Contents

**The Essence of the Organs** 23

# Imagine...

...our body was quite different to what we had always perceived it to be. Let's assume our scientific knowledge of the human being was only a part of the truth and our organs were not only clusters of cells but also spiritual soul formations that were equipped with structures and functions for our existence on this planet. What would that mean for us – for our consciousness, for our body, for our health and for our striving towards a fulfilled life?

These questions, once we started asking them, elicited unconventional answers. Surprisingly, again and again parallels emerged to the words of mystics from history, to the findings of quantum physics and to the cellular communication through light. Finally we became aware of an enormous complexity of body and soul, which could no longer be discussed or understood in a purely factual way.

Another language was needed. Our organs resisted being presented as a sum of facts, functions or even bearer of problems; they wanted to be perceived as spiritual and physical base elements of our existence, as elemental beings. Moreover, they wanted to reveal themselves in their beauty and perfection. Our organs are tired of us remembering them only in times of crisis or illness, where they have to direct our awareness to necessary changes. They would much rather help us to discover the magnificence of life and encourage us to celebrate our existence as unique beings every day anew.

This is how the portraits in this book emerged. They are portraits of the essences of our organs, portraits that want to touch us in their spiritual soul parts – an ode to life. They show us the perfection of existence and offer us an "update" to our understanding of the energetic functions of our organs. Perhaps the illustrations of the organ personalities will speak to you; maybe in between the lines you will discover one or two truths for yourself, or you might even perceive them simply as beautiful illustrations accompanied by lovely stories. In any case, we would like to invite you to see your organs differently and to appreciate the human body, including your own, more. Through this you just might discover more joie de vivre, better health and a new understanding of a way of being whole that comprises body – with all its organs – and soul.

# Preface

When in 2008 the book Reflexzonen und Organsprache (Reflexology and the Language of the Organ) was published I had taken a new step into spiritual psychosomatic medicine. The organs do not only want to admonish us and remind us to do something better or different; they have so much more to say to us. Above all, though, they want to reveal themselves to us in their infinite beauty and perfection. Thus I knew that my archetypal approach to the organs via stories and symbols could be no more than a beginning. Indeed, the essences of the organs have much deeper roots.

When a consciousness of spiritual and soul principles wants to manifest into reality it leads us through inspirations, coincidences and encounters. Thus in May 2009, during the authors' meeting celebrating twenty-five years of the publishing company Neue Erde, I met the painter Anne Heng. I already knew her wonderful paintings from The Tree Angel Oracle and so I put my request to her – that together we could present the organs as beings in words and pictures. She was immediately enthusiastic, and from that point on this work has been characterized by, and allowed to develop an unbreakable group of, "Us": the organs, Anne and me.

Our organs want to be perceived as spiritual and physical base elements of our existence, as elemental beings.

At the Frankfurt Book Fair in autumn 2009, Andreas Lentz of Neue Erde publishing was the fourth person to join. This "Us" has been continuously enriched by further people: by Hilde

Fuhs with her translations of the organs into music from ancient sources; by Veronika Berkenhoff and Catrin Benecke with their inspired work on translating our contemplation of the organs into kinesiological terms; and by friends who have added to the alignment of the project with their thought-provoking input.

A further valuable contribution to the events was made by Walter von Holst and Sita Andrea, who offered their know-how and their experiences in the field of crystal healing.

For a long time as we worked on the book, when our friends asked exactly what these organ beings were we were not able to give a satisfactory answer. We were able to describe them though, which meant we could convey a fairly good impression of them. But several aspects of our explanations still remained cloudy. This changed instantly when we showed the paintings to our friends or had them read the texts. They all, without exception, responded by saying that the pictures and the words touched something within their soul.

This confirmed to us once more that we were on the right track. Admittedly, the organs did not always make it easy for us. There were times when we did not manage a single line nor a single brushstroke, when adverse winds prevented us from writing and painting, when everything seemed to be blocked. Then again, there were (fortunately) plenty of times when everything seemed to flow effortlessly, when word nestled next to word and where a painting seemed to create itself, beautifully, more or less by itself. These differing experiences were of course created, or at least enhanced, by how in touch with ourselves we were, how far we trusted our inner guidance and how much room we gave these elemental beings to exist and develop within our own inner worlds.

Our first work meeting in Anne's studio was powered by an enormous joy. Through our work, the beauty of the essence of the organs was finally being perceived and appreciated. Our next task was to transfer this appreciation into a visible and readable work of art.

We agreed that the spiritual beings of the organs would speak in first-person statements in order to best introduce and disclose themselves. We also realized that their personification could not serve as a vis-à-vis confronting the reader; instead, the beings of the organs want to invite the observer to tune in to their qualities and experience them directly. To facilitate tuning in to them more closely, the organs allowed us to depict them sometimes from the side and sometimes from behind. Thus was created a “pull” for the reader/viewer into the organs’ consciousness fields that lends the words and illustrations an even greater power.

We then decided which organs would be represented in the book and selected the corresponding text and pictures; this process was often accompanied by inner conflicts. Through all these examinations of the deep inner processes we had gained the insight that we as humans are able to sense and experience the essence of the organs, that it is possible to describe and paint them. But there remained still something that worked on the mind but that was not tangible, something that we could not label.

We finally realized that this is actually the most profound part of our whole project. Our mind is just not able to access this level of existence. Now, after finalizing the first selection of organs, we feel confident in agreeing with what a dear friend, Gottfried Hermann, said: that it was not us who created the illustrations and texts but that our task consisted in providing the organs with a means of expression. This did all happen through us, but it was not us who brought it into being. This also explains why every time we pick up the illustrations or the manuscript we are amazed all over again.

We wish you much joy, health and a life of being in harmony with your organs.

Anne Heng and Ewald Kliegel
Weilburg and Stuttgart

# Introduction

*The body is the translator of the soul into the visible.*

CHRISTIAN MORGENSTERN[1]

# Orientation Towards the Healing Field

"The languorous hush of the organs" – that is how H. G. Gadamer defined health.[2] However, healing moves beyond this. Beyond the absence of physical and psychological discomforts, "being whole" is an experience or a state of being in which we are in touch with our deepest inner being. It is a lifelong process with many paths and one of these paths touches on the body and its organs. With what they have to tell us they enrich us: with self-respect, with the discovery of our potential, with a wonderful inner attunement and, of course, also with health.

However, it is not those 1.5 kilos of liver tissue or the 140 grams of the pancreas alone that offer us these gifts. For this we can give thanks to the elemental beings of the organs, the fields of consciousness, that as spiritual essence guard our organs and the inner streams of information and energies on all physical, as well as soul, levels.

In our habitual thinking we forget far too easily that everything in the body works cooperatively, that the same blood provides nourishment for the tips of the toes as well as the roots of the hair and that all nooks of our body are linked through the autonomic nervous system, which embraces a length of about ten circumferences of the earth.

Furthermore, we live with the notion that occupying ourselves with that which is lacking or disturbed and not functioning is the only way in which health and healing works. But our body does not work like a steam engine, where we operate a valve and then the part that we expect to move does so. We are a complex system of body and soul in which linear modes of thought and simple mechanisms of cause and effect will bring us no success; in which such simplistic models just do not suffice. This is also exactly where modern medicine reaches its limits, since it consistently excludes the mental–spiritual needs of our being.

> The World in which we live is not the vale of tears that keeps us away from the summits of the divine; it is the bridge that connects us with it. We just have to bring light to the fogs of consciousness that prevent us seeing it.[3]

The elemental beings invite us to shift our perspective and to experience our organs differently. Freed from a purely material way of thinking, in this mode we can understand and orient ourselves towards the healing field of life. This mode is nothing like thinking, as we usually know it; it's more a holistic perceiving, sensing, observing – experiencing!

If we can connect with an organ's essence, a seed in us that we have neglected for far too long begins to regerminate. With its growth a basic knowledge of the spiritual roots of the organs unfolds, a consciousness that teaches us a renewed mindfulness for our body, and through this mindfulness – once it fully blossoms – we find our very own inner life force.

If we follow this invitation of the elemental beings we arrive at a dialogue with the deep levels of our being. In this we activate the spiritual blueprints of the organs and thus access, so to speak, the "updates" to our spiritual "organ software". Thus we arrive at a deeper appreciation of our body. This is an essential ingredient for our good health.

The elemental beings invite us to shift our perspective and to experience our organs differently.

Nevertheless, this does not mean to disregard medicine or neglect naturopathy. The knowledge about the nature of the organs that we would like to convey in this book is no simple new healing method that promises us health and a long life. We cannot condense it into pills and take it occasionally or when needed. It is more a way of getting in touch with ourselves and the forces inherent in us.

When we consider the human being in his or her entirety as a physical-spiritual unity, all healing methods have their place. Then every health trade or skill becomes an art of healing. With our awareness of the elemental beings of our organs we open up spiritual spaces in our consciousness, spaces for new things to happen. This can lead to miracles – although we should not actively expect them.

It would be just as wrong to hope for our rheumatism, stomach ulcers or cancer to be healed. All these illnesses are complex processes that we cannot "defeat" but only put in order, in tune with ourselves and our inherent nature. What medicine and individuals mostly focus on at present though is managing the disturbances and problems of health conditions – the symptoms. In this we do not allow enough room for the self-healing properties that we all possess.

If we open ourselves to the nature of our organs, we can change our attitude and find an inner equilibrium through which we can balance the stresses of our existence. This balance is what we generally call "health". Furthermore, on this path that also includes spiritual exploration, a state of "being whole" can unfold, since through opening up to the elemental beings of the organs we get in touch with the basic levels of our being. In such a connection we experience "being at home" in our body as much as in our soul. Sometimes we feel the spiritual soul fields of the organs' elemental beings directly. Then we perceive them as something like an angel – we are filled with a bright flowing – or we experience our body as the origin of pure joy.

With our awareness of the elemental beings of our organs we open up spiritual spaces in our consciousness, spaces for new things to happen. This can lead to miracles – although we should not actively expect them.

*Stop, where are you running?*
*Heaven is within you.*
*If you look for God elsewhere you miss him completely.*[4]

# Our Organs Invite Us

The nature of our organs points us in one direction: towards beauty and perfection of being. They align us with a form of healing that does not come from the outside but that is waiting for us inside of us. Our reasoned thinking has only very limited influence in this; that which is essential just cannot be grasped logically. Feelings and emotions are also considered by our mind to be vague, and they do not follow our will either. In another way though, these human levels are quite intelligible and clear.

With the nature of the organs it is similar. Here also we are confronted with a world that must appear very unorthodox to us as here we meet our fabric of soul and body outside our known patterns of thought. And still, it is exactly these unorthodox portals that we have to move through in order to find the creation forces of life. The elementals of the organs would like to encourage us to trust those qualities that are so often pushed into the background: sensitiveness, intuition, compassion, receptivity and the courage to really live all of this. With such a perspective, miracles and healings can occur.

A saying of the bushmen of the Kalahari Desert runs: "The human is like an ant that tries to extinguish the sun by peeing on it." We always want to be in control of everything and forget that we are a part of the universe and thus an integral part of it; that next to our will and desires there is another, more profound, inherent spiritual order that serves the great whole, the "all One".

In this context the depictions of the essence of the organs are something like a fragrance that wafts around our nose, as the aroma of the morning coffee reaches us. In order to experience this fragrance again and again we need some small assistance and memory aids. The following exercises serve as such; we can do them on a meditation cushion as well as in a crowded tram or in the middle of a flower field. The most essential thing is to allow our intents and our will to come to rest behind our thoughts. Often a few minutes suffice to create an inner space in which we can encounter the spiritual layers of our body.

Each of the following exercises is suited in a particular way to reach this inner space of calm. Sometimes we need a bit longer and at other times a few breaths are sufficient to create in us a readiness for equanimity. It is suggested

**Exercise 1 – The Energy Flow**

Seat yourself comfortably, feet firmly on the ground, and place your hand on your navel.

Now imagine your feet growing roots down into the earth.

With every breath that you feel through the rising and falling of your belly underneath your hands your roots keep spreading further and further into the earth.

Sometimes these roots reach so deep down into the core of the earth that they touch the magma. Allow your roots to joyfully splash about in the magma and observe how all wearying thoughts and feelings flow away into it.

Now move your attention to your crown area.

Imagine you are opening a spiritual sunroof up there and then select a beautiful star from the starry sky.

Allow this star to radiate down into you and feel how this pleasant light flows through your spine and through the tips of your roots into the magma.

With time this light starts to sparkle like a bubble bath around your roots. In this way, you form a beautiful connection between your outer universe and your inner earth, suffused with light; and you feel how good it is to be an intermediary for energies. With this you are firmly anchored in your place in the present moment.

Feel how through this connection all wearying energies drain off and are transformed. Give space to this flowing and simply listen to the voice of your elemental beings.

that you accompany the exercises with conscious breathing in and out.

The first exercise has proven value in connecting to the energy flows. This exercise "blows" through our system, in a manner of speaking, and activates the contact to our inner strength. With the second exercise, which originates in Zen Buddhism, we can clear our thoughts; then out of the unconscious background fields solutions can appear that we would never otherwise have thought of.

The third exercise is an example of an imaginary journey into our inner worlds. Through symbolically moving into the depth we experience support from our unconscious archetypal levels[5] and receive pointers for beneficial changes. After aligning to our inner impulses we can open up to an organ and its essence. For this we direct the focus of our attention to an organ principle. It does not matter whether we open the book as if "by chance", whether we purposefully engage with one particular organ or whether we are in the process of dealing with a physical, psychological or spiritual topic, or a soul topic.

**Exercise 2 – The Cloud Portal**

Imagine your thoughts were like clouds that move across the sky.

When you see such a thought cloud, greet it like a passing pedestrian.

Allow the thought to move on without holding on to it.

Do not let yourself be drawn into a dialogue with it either. If necessary this can happen later, but now is just not the time for it.

If you do not hold on to it the next thought cloud will also move on, and the next, and bit by bit you will start enjoying more and more of the empty blue sky inside yourself.

> *Oh! Valiantly heat the spirit with spirit and power / that it may become fiery and blazing. Even if thereby the delicate glass of the brain should burst.*[6]

**Exercise 3 – The Inner Lake**

Imagine you walk through a tranquil wood and reach a clearing with a spreading lake. Calm and inviting, it reflects the sun.

You follow the path in the woods down towards the water's edge and see that the path continues through the lake.

Somewhat hesitant, you make a first small step into the water and are surprised that neither your shoe nor your trousers get wet as an air film places itself around your foot and leg.

With the second foot also a pleasant freshness reaches you, which feels very good after the walk.

With each step you feel more secure; it is a sensation of being held.

Even when you reach the point where your mouth and nose dip under the surface of the water it is amazing – your breath flows yet more lightly and freely. It is as if the lake provides you with an additional energy reserve.

Next, with the change of perspective through your eyes, which are now under the water, a fascinating world opens up. It is the same woods as before, only richer in forms and colours, more intense as an experience, more luxuriant in the emotional world. The walk becomes a floating in beauty beyond words that amazes you and conveys a great joy to the depth of your soul.

Walking further you meet an organ in the shape of its essence that invites you to get to know its perfection and its characteristics.

You experience a familiarity with this representative of your body in connection with a comprehensive knowledge, a rediscovery of deepest soul qualities.

Furthermore, you make contact with an aliveness within you that you had nearly forgotten. Before you walk on, the representative of the organ leaves you a small present and directs you to the path upwards.

In your own timing and as it feels right for you, your steps turn again towards the surface of the water.

Now you look from below through the mirror of the lake and realize that the path upward moves on towards the sun. Moreover, you now clearly recognize your direction.

With each step the lake rolls off you again, and giving thanks to your soul you start walking this path, knowing full well that the lake will soon await you again with other valuable encounters.

# Retracing the Connection with the Organ's Essence

Through the inner connection with the elemental beings of the organ we retrieve the "ideal software" from the ether field into the structure of our body and soul. Now we only need to update this information in our cells and organs. For this we can call on persons with healing skills who can tune in to this information.

Equally, we can conduct this spiritual work ourselves. When we use the term "work", we are not talking about "doing" in the classical meaning but about an increased awareness with which we present our organs with a smile and with which we give thanks to the perfection that lives within us. The illustrations and the texts facilitate this work.

While the first-person narrative already allows us to sympathize with the organ and thus sense its magnificence, the illustrations offer us the possibility to merge with the organ principle. With this the organ beings invite us to experience all their information and energies directly. Furthermore, we achieve an inner fusion with the organ principle and emerge into an inner world that provides a healing field.

In order to establish a good connection with the essence of the organs we should always actively dedicate one whole day to one spiritual organ principle. For this we could, for example, extract a core sentence from the text and actively recall and reflect on this sentence at different points during the day: What does this sentence mean in the context of just this situation? – How can I improve my life now using this information?

This may seem to us a small step only but still, hereby we possibly receive an insight that helps us further, or out of it might come clarity about an upcoming decision.

The same applies to each of the illustrations. If we continue to hold them mentally or physically in front of our eyes we discover this and that detail, which in connection with the present situation highlight completely new perspectives and solutions. With such awareness, throughout the day we continuously update the calibration of our programmes with the perfection of the spiritual levels of the organs, and we join with the current of energies and information that flows in the depth of our soul.

In all this, we should always allow room for the question of how we can now use this inner presence of the organs' elemental beings to heal something in us.

In order to establish a good connection with the essence of the organs we should always actively dedicate one whole day to one spiritual organ principle.

How our mind evaluates the situation is not crucial. Much more important is that we feel as acutely as possible with our whole heart and let ourselves be guided by our intuition. Thus an impulse can, for example, when choosing the lunchtime meal, recommend a food combination that we otherwise would never have thought of. Another impulse can spontaneously direct our steps in another direction, it can gently prompt us at the next motorway exit to continue our journey through the countryside – despite an appointment – or to choose a route that we have never used before. At the same time, an inner impulse can animate us to speak to someone or to give more space to a meeting.

These impulses can concern comprehensive topics, like questions on the general overall design of the day, but also deal with nearly inconspicuous incidents like a smile that we give to someone. In any case the decision as to whether we surrender to an impulse should not depend on mental deliberations or be determined by time factors, but by scanning our emotions to ascertain whether we are in any way touched by this impulse.

An interesting possibility consists in drawing or painting a picture of an organ. For this we simply need to take a sketchbook and a pen or pencil of any colour, begin without any aim or concept and let ourselves be guided by our inner impulses. The artistic qualities of the work are not important here; what matters is how intensely we dedicate ourselves to doing this. For interpretation of what we produce we'd be best advised to let a day pass in order to gain "inner distance" when looking at the picture.

Another beautiful exercise for paying our respect to the organs consists in dedicating each day to a different organ. This is at the same time a spiritual spring-cleaning of the organs in the form of a mindful journey through the body. Since every journey follows a very personal route there is no determined sequence here either. We can select the organ of the day at random and identify it through tuning in to our body or according to a sequence that makes sense to us.

As an addition a diary of events can be useful, where every evening we record our feelings and emotions in "catchphrases". We are free to end the "organ day" with a positive conclusion in the form of a short sentence.

*Treat your body well so that your soul feels like living in it.*[7]

# Energetic Treatments Facilitate Contact

In order to anchor the beings of the organs even more in our body awareness we should prepare a field for them in which they are welcome. Suitable for this are all treatments that are also used for energetic harmonization. The old Chinese teachings say that we swim in a sea of energy like a fish in water; these are the energies to use. All cultures have found access to these and developed treatments accordingly. We know them variously as acupuncture points, meridians, chakras and reflex zones. They are the portals where we are most intensely in interaction with our surrounding energy fields and where we can particularly well receive impulses to contribute to inner regulation and harmony.

Even though such knowledge has, in the West, for many centuries been suppressed or disregarded, about 150 years ago a development started in the course of which Western practice too opened windows for these energetic treatments. In Western treatments, the portals where a special connection between the inner and the outer world exists are called the reflex zones. They are our "maps of health" onto which the organs project their conditions and where we can convey our treatment impulses towards the inner world – to the organs.

The most familiar reflex zones are those on the feet. In many ancient cultures foot massage is part of that culture's traditional alternative medicine. Today we know of more than thirty reflexology systems[8]: On the hands, on the ears, on the back, on the face and on the cranium. For accessing the essence of the organs we can in principle use all of them, though those on the hands and feet have proven of particular value for energetic attunements. Skin, connective tissue and blood do not have any fixed correlation with reflex zones. As a general application for these organs we can massage the elbows and hollows of the knees. These areas require particular attention with regard to the intensity of the touch. Here we should run our hands over the skin only very gently.

As already pointed out, essential for all of these treatments is not the amount of pressure but how closely connected on an inner level we are with the other person. Since reflex zones are energetic phenomena it is not surprising that those methods that influence the body in a similar way offer the best support in regulating the physical and spiritual/soul functions of the organs. Light, colours, essential oils and crystals are particularly supportive and effective.

> *Thus God allowed neither the beauty nor the potency of crystals to vanish but wanted them to be appreciated and praised and to serve as a remedy on earth.*[9]

# Crystal Massages and Reflexology – The Golden Paths

Integrating crystal massage into energetic systems offers a wonderful opportunity to intensify our access to the essence of the organs. To this end we may first identify the area on the feet or hands with the help of the reflexology chart. Then we search this area with either the finger or a quartz crystal wand, moving in gentle circles and searching the maximum reference point. This is the point where we feel the most intense reaction.

This search is mostly effected through a nearly imperceptible touch, a brushing over the area. By no means is this supposed to be painful or even uncomfortable. When we massage someone else's hands or feet, the maximum reference point can show itself through an obvious change in the person's breathing. Doing it ourselves, we often register the maximum reference point in the form of feelings, pictures or bodily sensations. There can also be surprising perceptions. A sensation of lightness might register with us, for example; or we might feel absolutely whole on an inner level; a grounding heaviness might come up; it can be joyful or full of relish, or there might also be sad or angry feelings.

No matter which quality comes out, every intense sensation shows us that we are in touch with the spiritual soul principle of an organ.

Once we have reached that point we do not have to do anything to start with but just stay there calmly without movement for three breaths and dedicate ourselves mentally to the essence of the organ. The tangible point serves hereby as a body anchor that we can touch again and again in order to establish contact in our awareness with the corresponding elemental being. After about five conscious activations of three breaths in length each via this body anchor the inner connections will be firmly stored. Then they can be called forward again at any time through simply touching these zones.

# Our Great Helpers: Minerals and Crystals

Crystals are particularly effective as, owing to their crystal structure, they are in intense resonance with the organs and their elemental beings. The wise ones of our ancestors' societies were of the opinion that each tiny part of the universe is animated and ensouled, and that everything is filled with spirit and sound. In this they anticipated the insight of modern quantum physics.

This principle applies even more emphatically to the world of minerals and crystals that prove these abilities in many technical applications. The best-known example for this is the focusing and amplifying of light quanta through crystals with lasers; but our information era is based on the silicon crystal. The ability of crystals to direct the current of quanta is responsible for this. And if we take only one small step further from here we have to grant the quanta consciousness, following the insights of the great physicists of the twentieth and twenty-first centuries.

We may also assume such a consciousness for crystals. Furthermore, crystals constitute beings with consciousness that help us to tune into the essence of our organs. For this interaction we on earth are provided with an abundance of crystals that thus serve us as translators of the spiritual impulses into the soul level and further into the physical. The following chart names for each organ being two crystals that are a particularly good match to the respective organ principle. For this selection I offer much gratitude to Walter von Holst and Sita Andrea and their understanding of crystals' elemental

The wise ones of our ancestors' societies were of the opinion that each tiny part of the universe is animated and ensouled, and that everything is filled with spirit and sound.

beings in crystal healing.

Should though another crystal, one not in the chart, suggest itself to us, then this one is definitely the right one to use. Then we can look up the crystal's properties in one of the many available crystal-healing guidebooks to discover which aspect of an organ principle attempts to find its way through this crystal into consciousness and into our life.

The crystal that we have chosen or that has chosen us will further enhance our awareness for the corresponding essence of the organs. We can carry the appropriate crystal with us as a drum stone or pendant over the time when we are working with the organ. Furthermore, we can place the crystals on the reflex zones and also massage the vital body (otherwise known as the subtle body) in the area above the organ as well as on the reflex zones.

Michael Gienger describes this type of massage in his book Crystal Massage for Health and Healing[10] as follows:

> Vital body massage concentrates on treating the whole person at the energetic level, rather than treating the physical body alone. The massage consists of a very gentle touching of the skin, with the intention of harmonizing and vitalizing the energy field that encircles and penetrates the body. This field is also called the etheric body, the vital aura, the morphic field, the subtle body or the vital body.

This massage is purely intuitive; the direction as well as the intensity of the skin contact is carried out by tuning in to how to go about it in the present moment. If we surrender to this with our whole heart, then the deeper layers of our consciousness will take over and guide us as we use these treatments.

**Correlation of Healing Crystals with the Organs**

| Organ | Crystal | Affirmation |
|---|---|---|
| Bladder | Halite | I open and close, I confine and I surrender. |
| | Sodalite | I defend my values with loyalty. |
| Blood | Rhodonite | I carry the raw material of life and healing within me. |
| | Hematite quartz | I seize life with my inspired will. |
| Brain | Diamond | I control spirit, soul and body. |
| | Tansanite | I convey meaningful perspectives. |
| Connective tissue | Klinoptilolite | I hold, nourish and renew all structures of life. |
| | Alabaster | I save and preserve the structures in their place. |
| Ears | Cavansite | I accept my own importance. |
| | Larimar | Here and Now I follow the inner call to myself. |
| Eyes | Polychrome tourmaline | I convey the world as colour and idea. |
| | Disthene | I see things as they are. |
| Feet | Basalt | I am rooted in the ultimate source of existence. |
| | Landscape jasper | I build on experiences and am linked with the path of my life. |
| Gall bladder | Azurite | I dissolve spiritual patterns and define. |
| | Zirconite | I remove disturbances and stay the course. |
| Hands | Lapis lazuli | In dignity I follow the impulses of the spirit. |
| | Mookaite | Playfully I create reality. |
| Heart | Rubin | I am strong in my rhythm and seize life. |
| | Danburite | With loving sensitivity I establish connections. |
| Hips | Granate | I am the tireless engine. |
| | Chiastolite | I focus and connect extremes. |

| | | |
|---|---|---|
| Intestine, large | Stromatolite<br>Sapphire | I allow and make the best of it.<br>I focus on the essential. |
| Intestine, small | Carneol<br><br>Vesuvianite | Self-assured, I reach for what is good for me.<br>I choose what is suitable and decode it. |
| Kidneys | Nephrite<br>Nuummite | I filter the living out of the stream.<br>I am the ancient force of the ancestors. |
| Knee | Sardonyx<br><br>Biotite lens | Determined and dignified, I implement what needs doing.<br>I stand for perseverance and springy elasticity. |
| Liver | Chrome Diopside<br><br>Malachite | I creatively strengthen all life processes with vigour.<br>I draw from the abundance of pictures and from imagination. |
| Lungs | Blue topaz<br>Blue coral | I absorb, I release and I let flow.<br>I take part and allow everyone to partake. |
| Mammary gland | Amber<br>Mangano-calcite | I am the nourishing mother.<br>I bring prosperity and growth. |
| Nose | Seraphinite<br><br>Rhodochrosite | I seize the opportunity with sure instinct.<br>I dance sensuously. |
| Pancreas | Brazilianite<br><br>Imperial topaz | I cushion imbalances and satisfy the shortage.<br>I am generous abundance. |
| Reproductive organs, female | Pink opal<br>Hydrogrossular | I playfully enjoy every moment.<br>I open up with the strength of the depth. |
| Reproductive organs, male | Thulite<br><br><br>Rubin zoisite | Strengthened by the power of the ancestors, I stand for the essence of being a man.<br>I give stability and self-confidence in the union. |

| | | |
|---|---|---|
| Shoulders | Hypersthene<br>Fluorite | I centre and carry the responsibility.<br>I broaden my boundaries. |
| Skin | Achate<br>Rose quartz | I protect layer by layer.<br>I sense, warmly and lovingly. |
| Spine | Selenite<br>Aegirine | I conduct light and peace.<br>I am flexible and give support. |
| Spleen | Charoite<br>Chrysobery | I throw out what interferes.<br>I transilluminate and monitor everything. |
| Stomach | Citrine<br>Sunstone | I transform conflicts into nourishment for the soul.<br>I am the loving Yes to existence. |
| Teeth | Sphen<br>Eudialyte | I bear everything and struggle through.<br>I fight for my survival. |
| Throat | Chalcedony<br>Turquoise | I communicate and explain.<br>I strengthen self-expression and facilitate acceptance. |
| Thymus | Heliotrope<br>Aquamarine | I define and preserve form.<br>I dynamically follow my destiny. |
| Thyroid | Fire opal<br>Libyan desert glass | I ignite the fire of enthusiasm.<br>I am the genius of the moment. |

# The Essence of the Organs

# Bladder

"District border capital" – that is how the Chinese people from ancient times onwards have characterized me, since it is in me that the energies for defence flow together. This is where they are at the disposal of body and soul, in order to protect from damaging influences.

Furthermore, I control the energetic functions at the border of our being where I can purposefully direct, contain or release the streams at the energy layers. People mostly feel this as the current of warmth that I send round the body from the feet to high up in the head.

In my connection to the soul levels I stabilize with this stream the defences of the being. From this grows a trust in the powers of self-respect, in the ability to hold a good basic tension and through all this to preserve a loving softness.

Letting go belongs to my being, as well as strength through inner flow. The clarity of insight emerging through these qualities opens the locks of compassion, awakens the powers of the movements of the mind and promotes dedication to gratitude for the soul awakening.

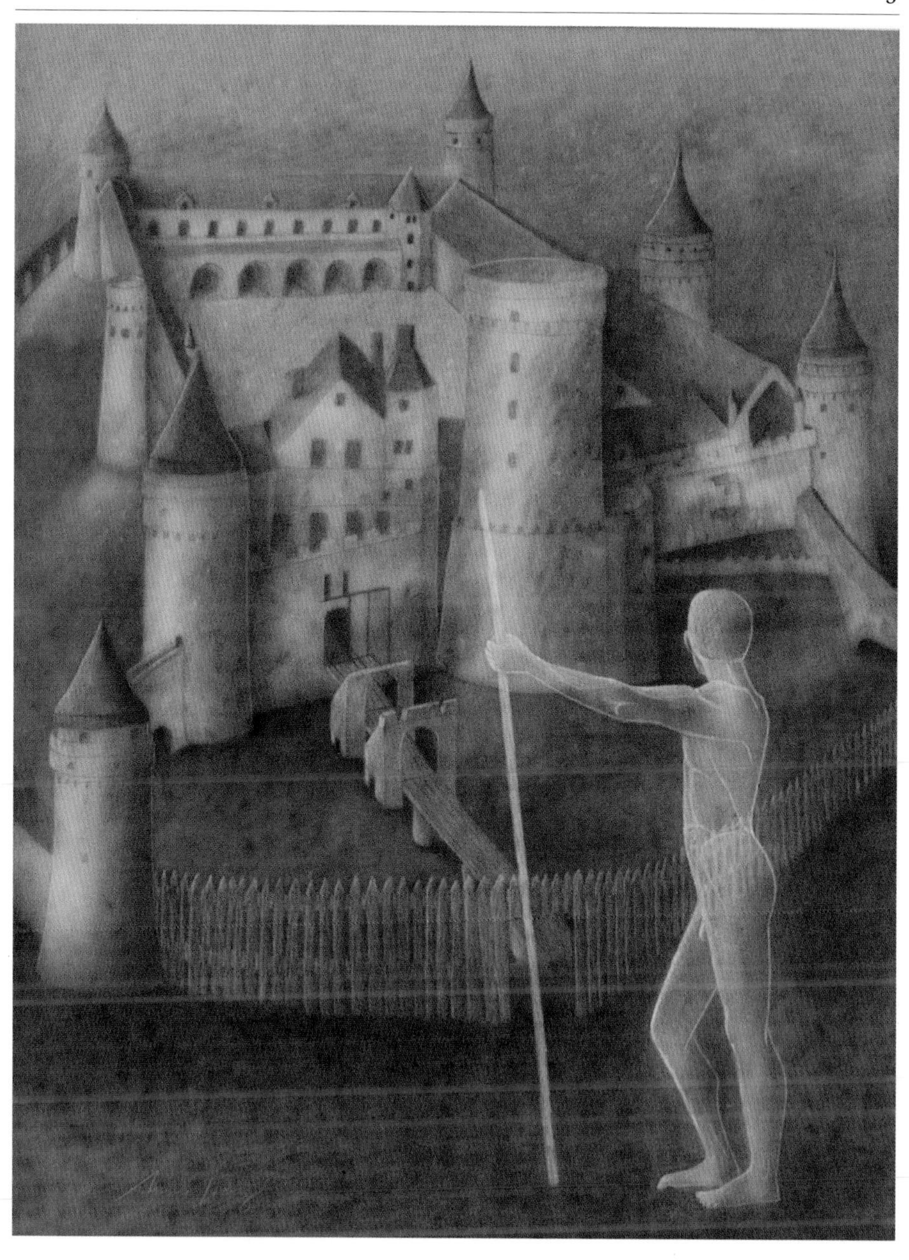

# Blood

I am the grail of the life energy and the liquid elixir that flows through it. Continuously pulsing, my red life force flows through the nearly unending meander of the body. From the fountain of my being I thus replenish over and over again a delta full of the finest vessels, which reach even the most distant corners of existence in order to provide the inner as well as the outer universe with energy and warmth.

The backflow I use to carry all burdens along and transform them into the basis for the power of the world that supplies us with the elixir of life. In this way, I complete the eternal cycle of being.

Ice-cold or simmering hot, my essence is a perfect mirror of the feelings that stir up a human being's blood out of the innermost depths of themselves. By virtue of the dynamics of these emotions I am the movement itself that runs with the flow of life, which fierily consumes itself and renews itself again and again.

Where I am is life in all its abundance, is the fountain of the freely flowing joy, is love in all its energy forms, is healing and salvation in the stream of existence.

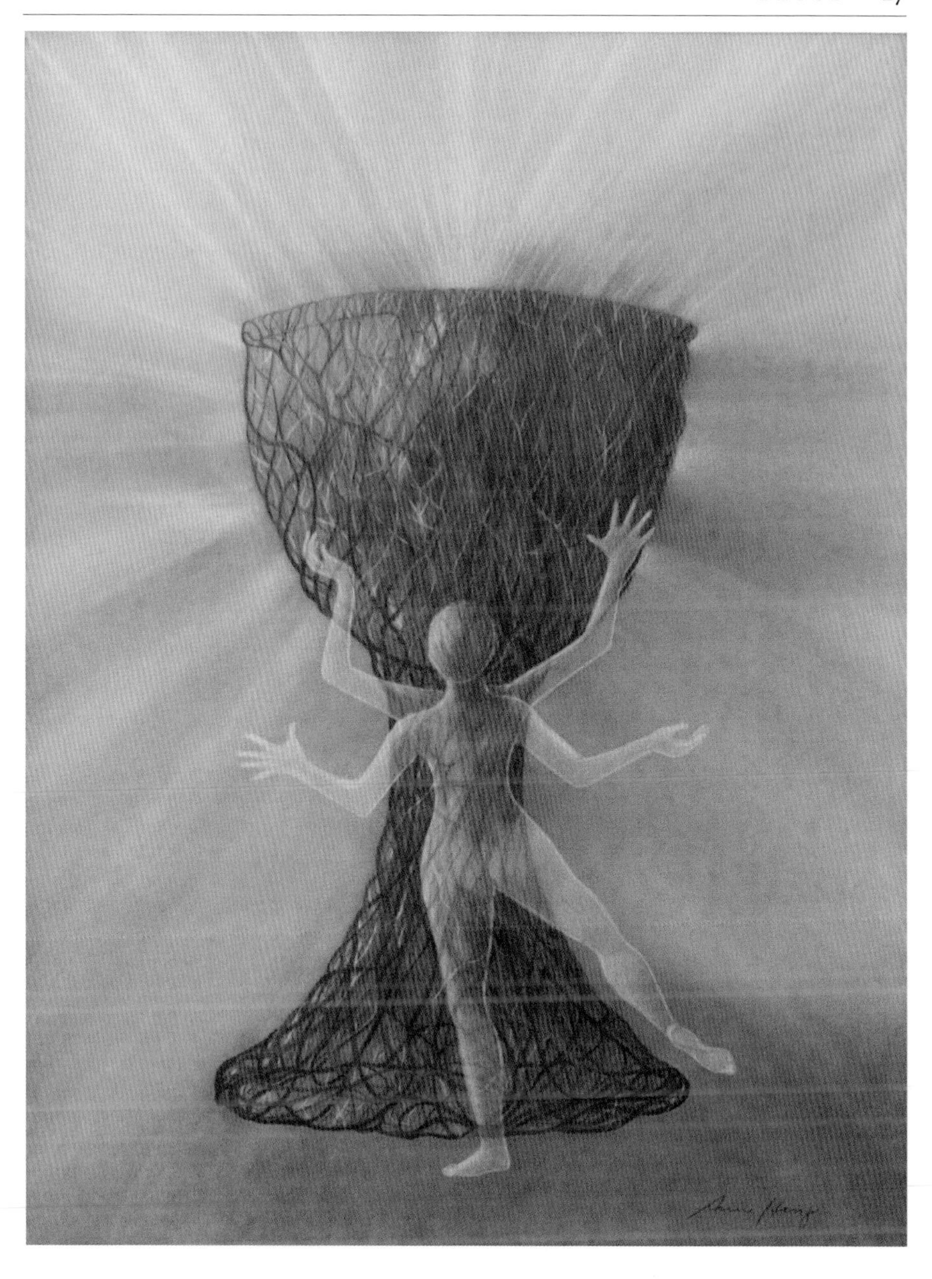

## Brain

Is it not wonderful: Each of my two halves contains its own world. While the left one is more devoted to the mind and logical thinking, the right one shines in the colours of emotions and intuition.

Jointly they create at every moment a new universe that is filled with love. Therein, through my interwoven spaces and dimensions, radiate the emotions and thoughts, in order to then receive their joint place in my unlimited ocean of perceptions.

I organize the inner coordination of the organs and look after their relationship to the outside world. Thereby I secure the person's survival on this planet and the opportunity for them to fill their life with experiences.

Essentially my task consists in sorting through everything and taking decisions accordingly. The results I then impart to the consciousness.

One of my greatest achievements consists in developing an identity or an "I am". This "I am" conveys to the human being a personality and the security of a self-awareness that enables assessments.

I am doing best when these assessments are constantly questioned and the person remembers with humour that all this can also be an illusion, as ultimately I simply mirror the person's very personal universe.

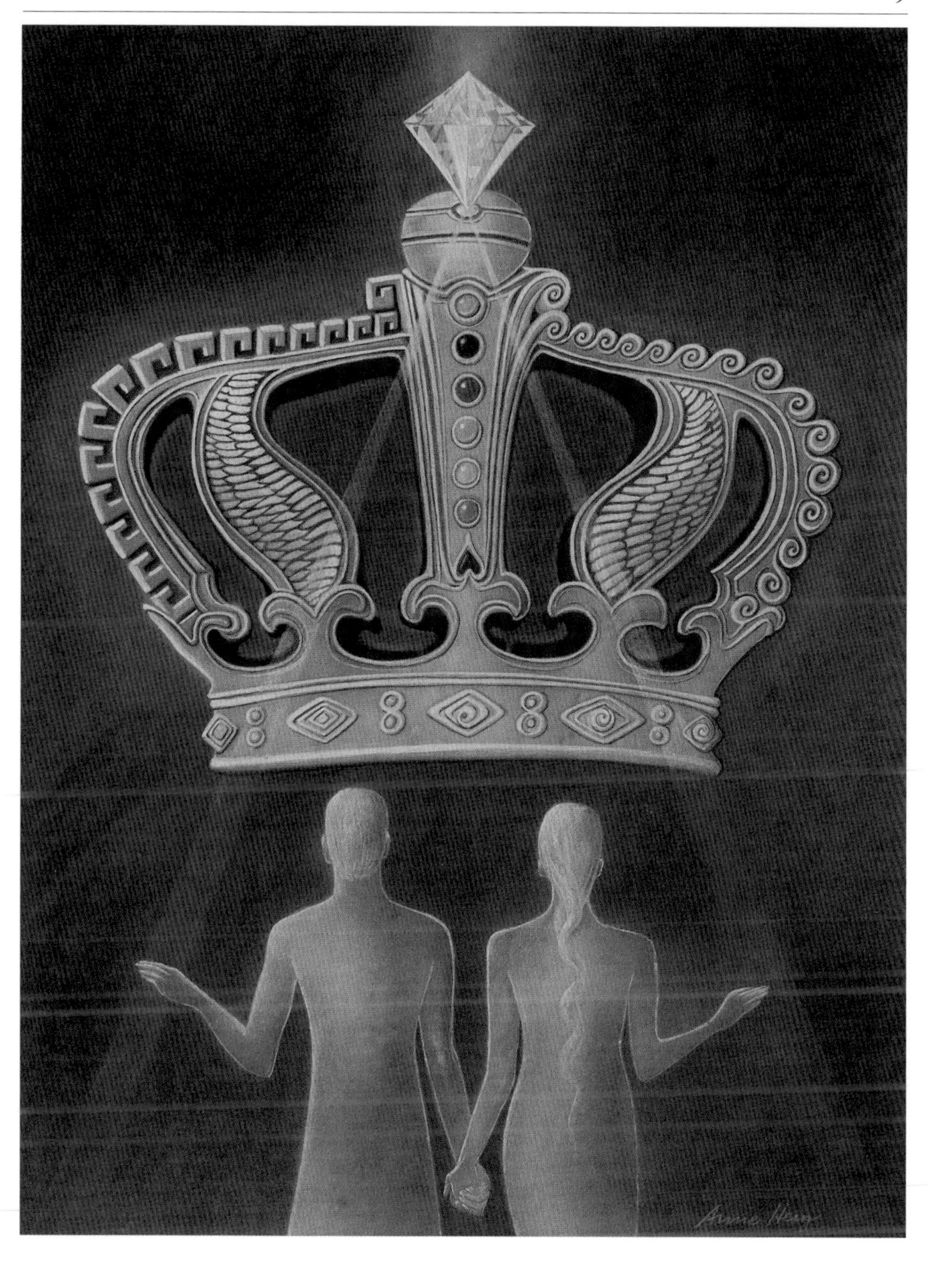

# Connective Tissue

For millions of years the rivers of life pulsate in my ocean. Here I provide a home for the cells, nourish them, look after their space and protect them. Pervaded by the light of the cells, I offer them a fluid clarity for communication and attunement on the highest level. In this, I take effect within a love that, in appreciation and engagement, again and again brings to the fore the joy in life, and also balances out adversities.

One of my most exquisite characteristics is my almost unlimited adaptability with which I am capable of transforming, modifying or newly designing everything. This becomes particularly apparent with physical or psychological trauma; when wounds need to be closed, when it is necessary to build up scar tissue and subsequently dissolve it again.

Ultimately I strive to become increasingly more diaphanous and flow freely with the stream of experiences. For this I need "alive food" that truly nourishes body and soul in its naturalness; that is a blessing for the person and that recognizes my nature. Thereby I succeed in transforming limitations into abilities and promoting the insight that all living can only persist in relationships of integrity.

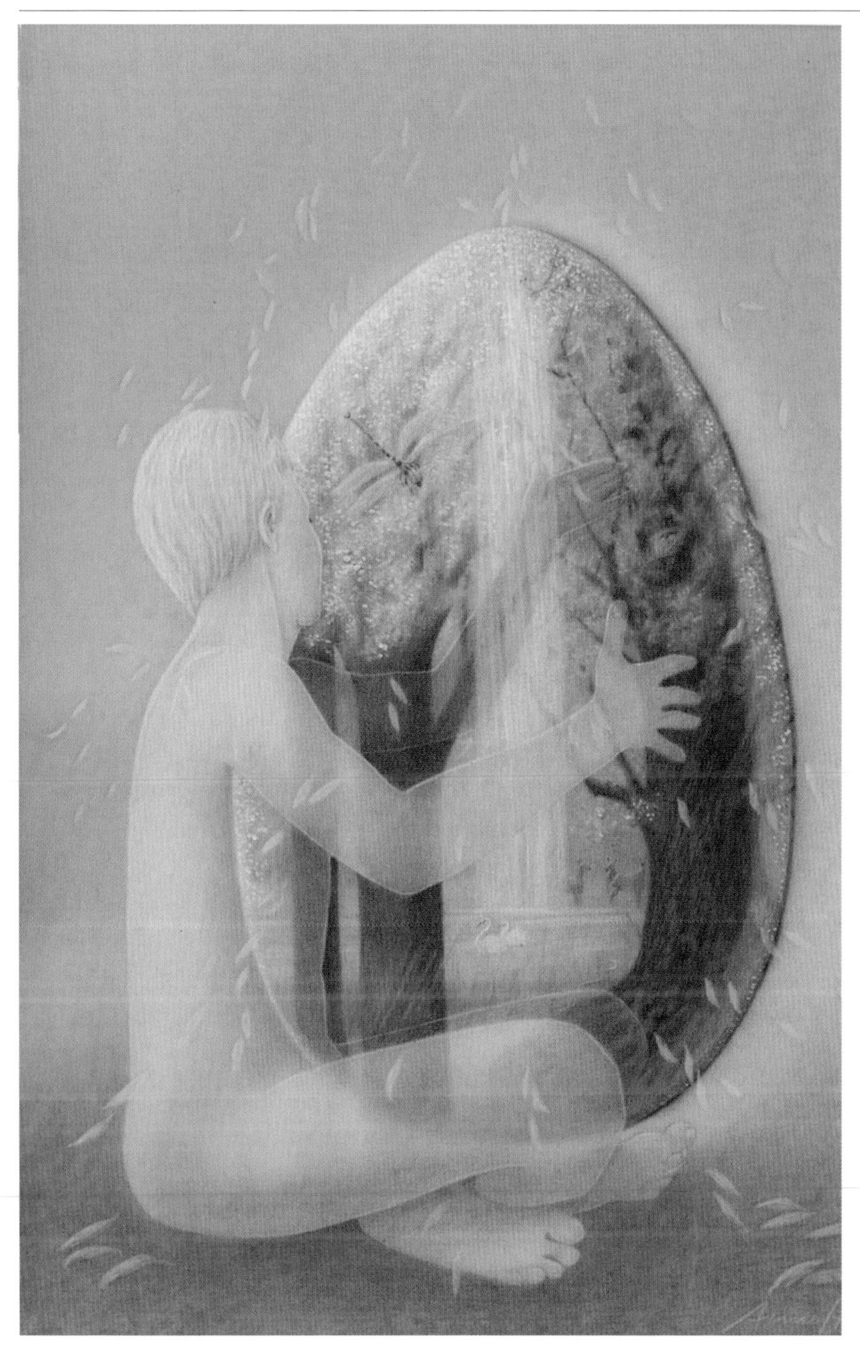

## Ears

Atoms, molecules, planets or galaxies: Everything resonates, sounds, sings and vibrates. The world is sound and we are the gates to the great orchestra of the universe.

In this we are particularly dedicated to the rhythms of our earth. We attune body and soul to them and provide a very personal speed in life, for a good balance between work and relaxation, for leisure that finds itself aligned with love, and for an openness that gives meaning to the inner voice's call for the life task, the vocation.

We are a part of the eternal stillness that reaches us when we allow ourselves to be touched by the music of a meadow filled with flowers. We are the perfect silence that captures us in the midst of a thunderous waterfall and we present for hearing the innermost sounding of the self that is awakened through alignment with the sound of the worlds.

We hold the inner balance between belonging to the all One and the very personal impulses a person has for their individual soul. Through this we can gift the person with the certainty that he or she is an indispensible part of the whole; and, more, that only through our individual belonging in all our love can the universe be whole.

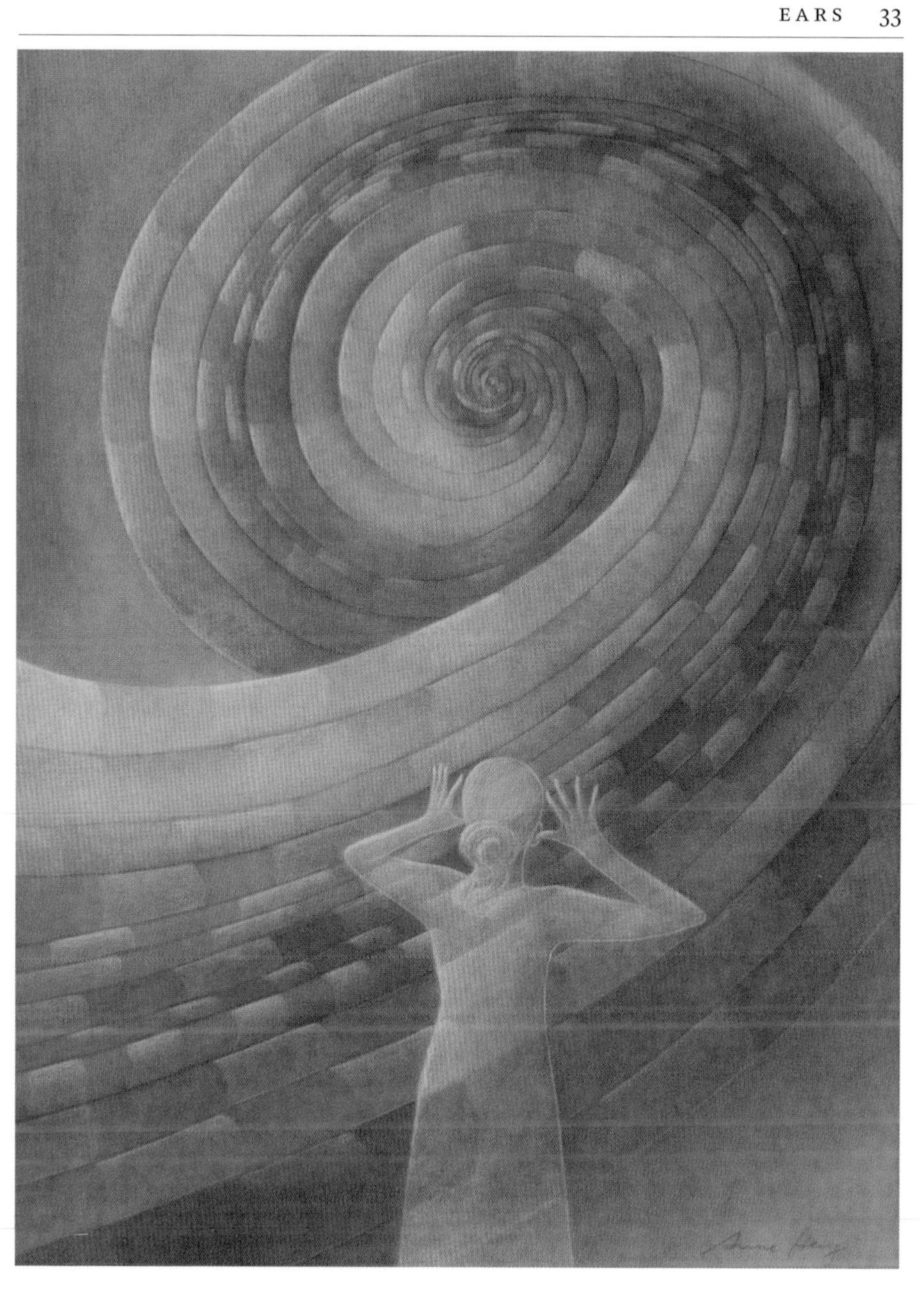

# Eyes

We convey that which is visible in the world towards the inner and guide the feelings through the gaze towards the outer. We allow the light spark of the universe to dance in our eyes and illuminate the world of the mind with the glow of emotions.

With the colours' rainbow we form space for pictures that fill with infinite thoughts and meanings. Passions, fears and joys flow through these "picture scopes", sprout, swell and ebb away. Adventures, experiences and longings complete all this to make inner pictures from which, each moment, we form a new world and fill in the supposedly missing.

More often than not we show the known. In those moments, however, in which people open up to our creative eyes they encounter the Now in all its facets. These moments, these gazes of the eyes, comprise of a deep contentment, a compliance with the knowledge that the world is whole and that uplifting beauty exists everywhere.

Compassionate and open-hearted, with our inner light we give happy moments of love in which we inspire people and things towards the beautiful – and awaken the view for a beauty which reveals insights into the coherence of life.

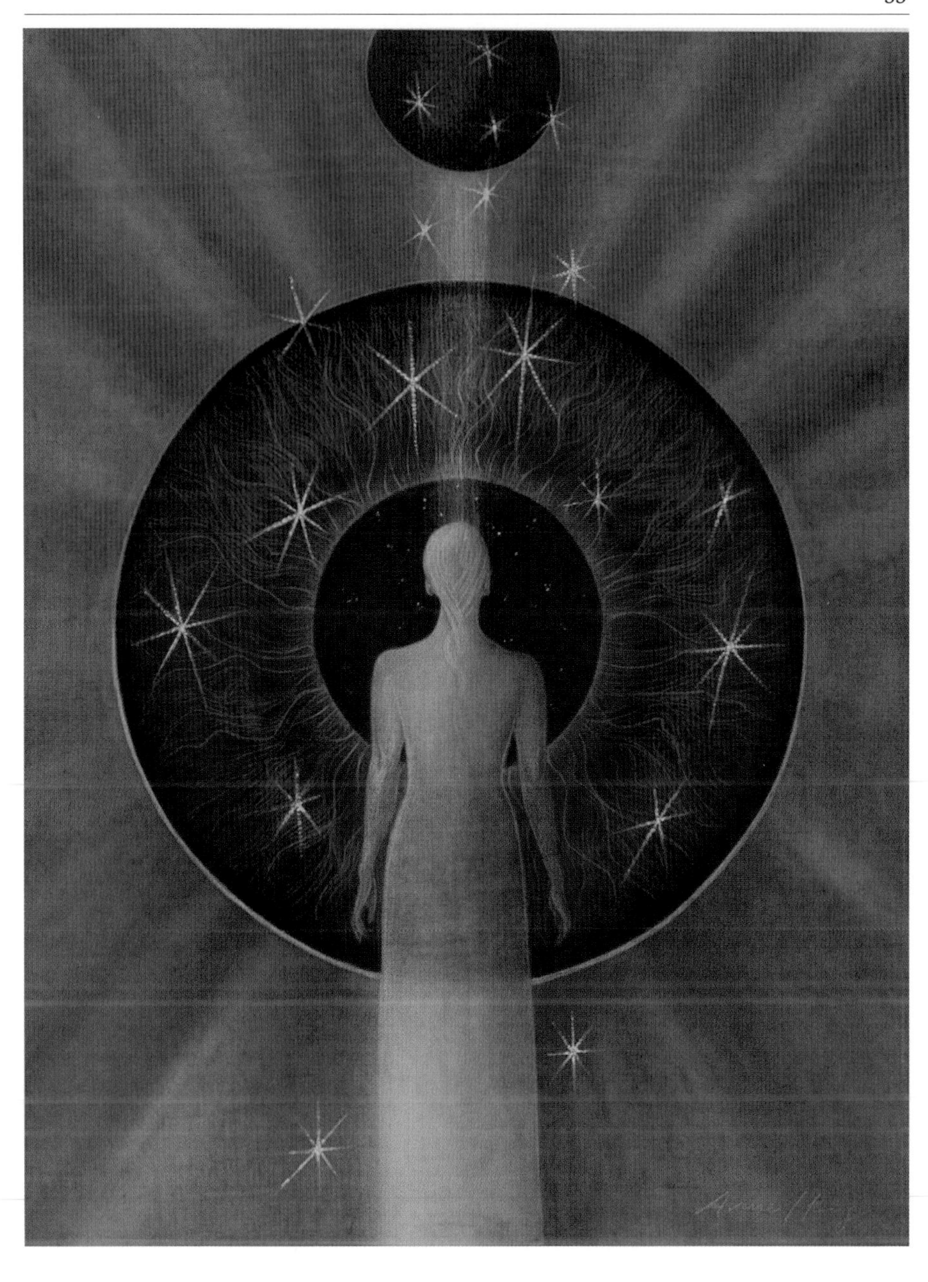

## Feet

Whether standing, walking or running: Our fine perceptions are the basis for contact with the earth. We do not only maintain an upright posture within the terrestrial gravity field, we also provide the person with roots in the world soul. We afford sturdiness in the storms of life, and we convey stability for increased balance and poise.

In proceeding we conquer spaces, let the world approach and at the same time move body and soul towards their goals.

Thereby it might appear at times as if the lightness of life has us float, while another time we need our inner orientation lights in order to move forward on viable paths.

The direction is right when we feel the connection to the great spiritual root system. Then our speed is also consistent with the development of the soul.

The mind is very surprised by some of these paths: thus we sometimes have the impression that despite our progress we are back at square one. If, however, we look closely we will recognize that through experiences on the way we have gained a better contact with the roots of life, and that ultimately we have always been at the finishing line anyway as every step includes the act of arriving already.

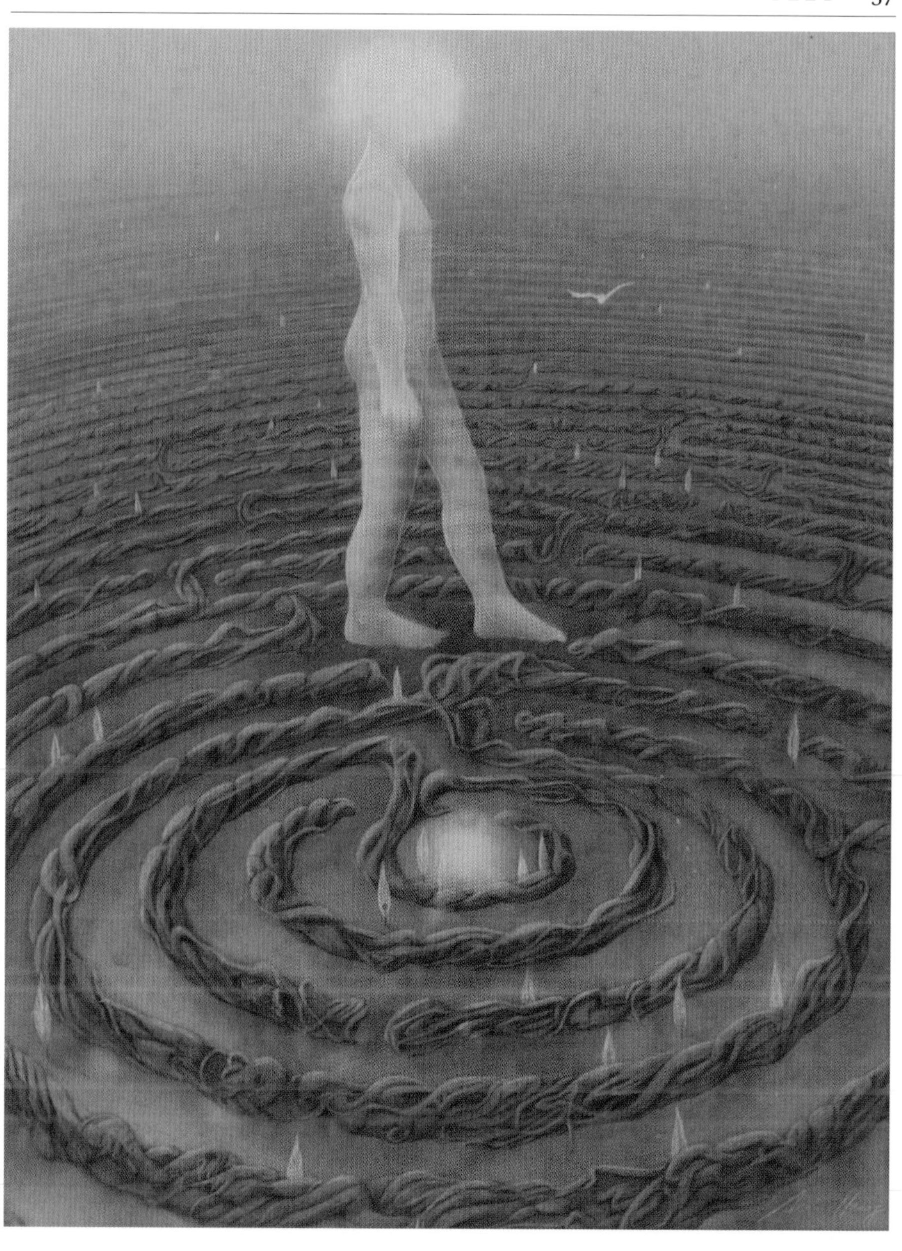

# Gall bladder

The bile that I store and release corresponds exactly to my being: As representative of inner guidance I resolve situations and lead to a pervading purity. Just as my essence separates the pure from the impure during the digestion process, I bring light to the emotions, thought patterns and behaviours.

Through this a linear striving gathers momentum – it leads beyond duality to clarity and allows for common-sense reasoning powers, even in the presence of crossing influences. Mostly, I am perceived as a primal trust that is pervaded by the light of compassion. Thus my knowing humbleness guarantees circumspect decisions that follow a clear life purpose.

In courageous self-confidence I can thus dissolve even those blockages that have been created through thoughts. My spiritual presence in stillness is permeated by a deep passion and love for life. This enables me to create a joyful ecstasy that spreads spontaneous outbreaks of joie de vivre and is even able to heal hatred.

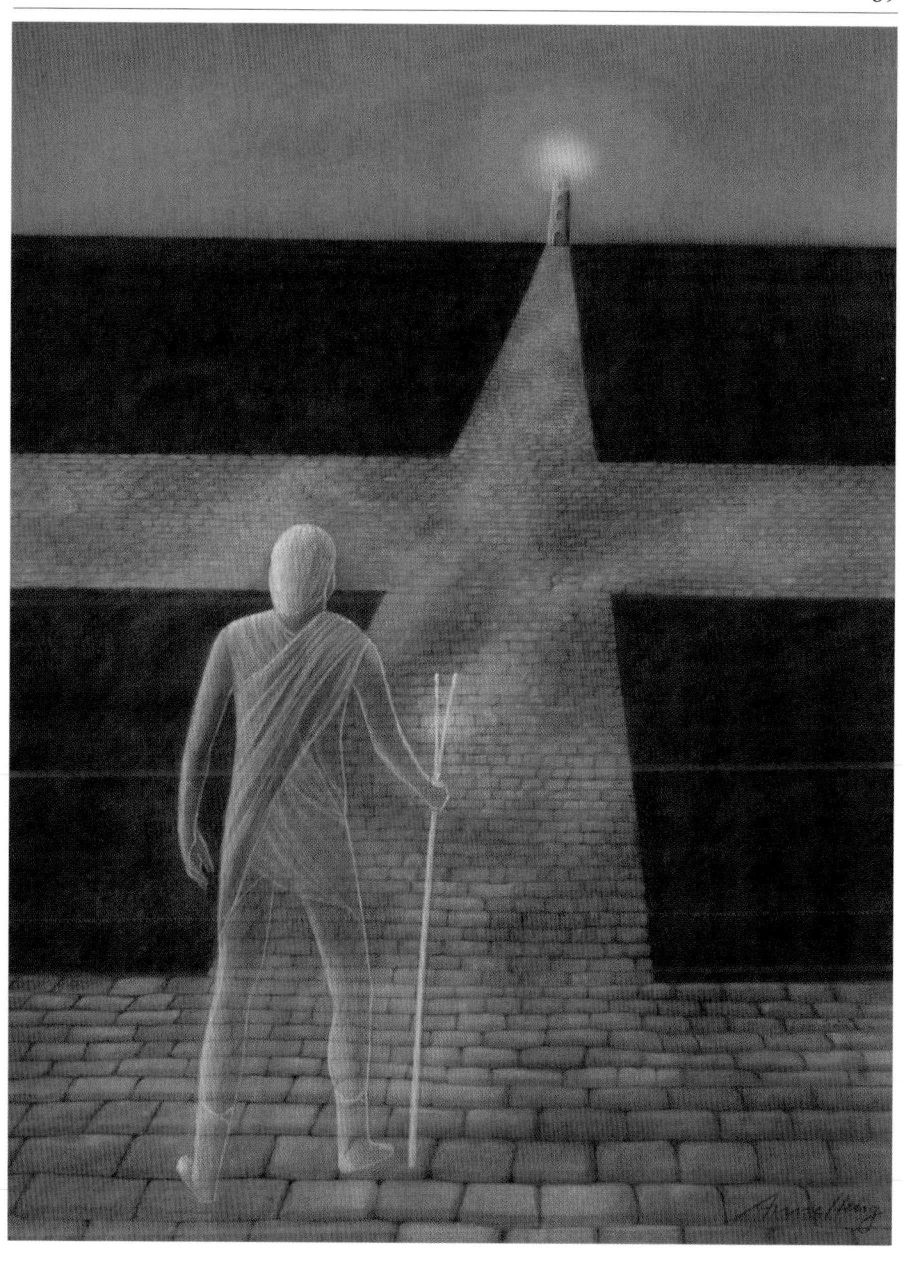

## Hands

We treat thoughts and feelings as if they exist in a tangible way. This is our basis for igniting the fire of ideas in order to advance life. We can sense even the finest energies around this and at the same time tackle things energetically.

We are the jugglers who mediate between spirit and matter, and through us the human is bound to the elements. Thus our task is to create facts out of spiritual energies and translate that which has been created into the language of spirit, to direct energies and to shape the game of life in both the material and the spiritual worlds.

In doing this we establish a trellis of relationships between everything alive. With us the person can rise above matter, and through us he or she is embedded in it.

We provide the support that is necessary for life, and through us the person is also held in the world. In our other aspect, we act through opening our hands. Generosity, releasing the obsolete and accepting what is available – with open hands we thus bring a deeply sensed dignity into all relationships. In such an appreciation we can serve as tools of love for the creation of a world in which human achievements continue to grow for everyone's benefit.

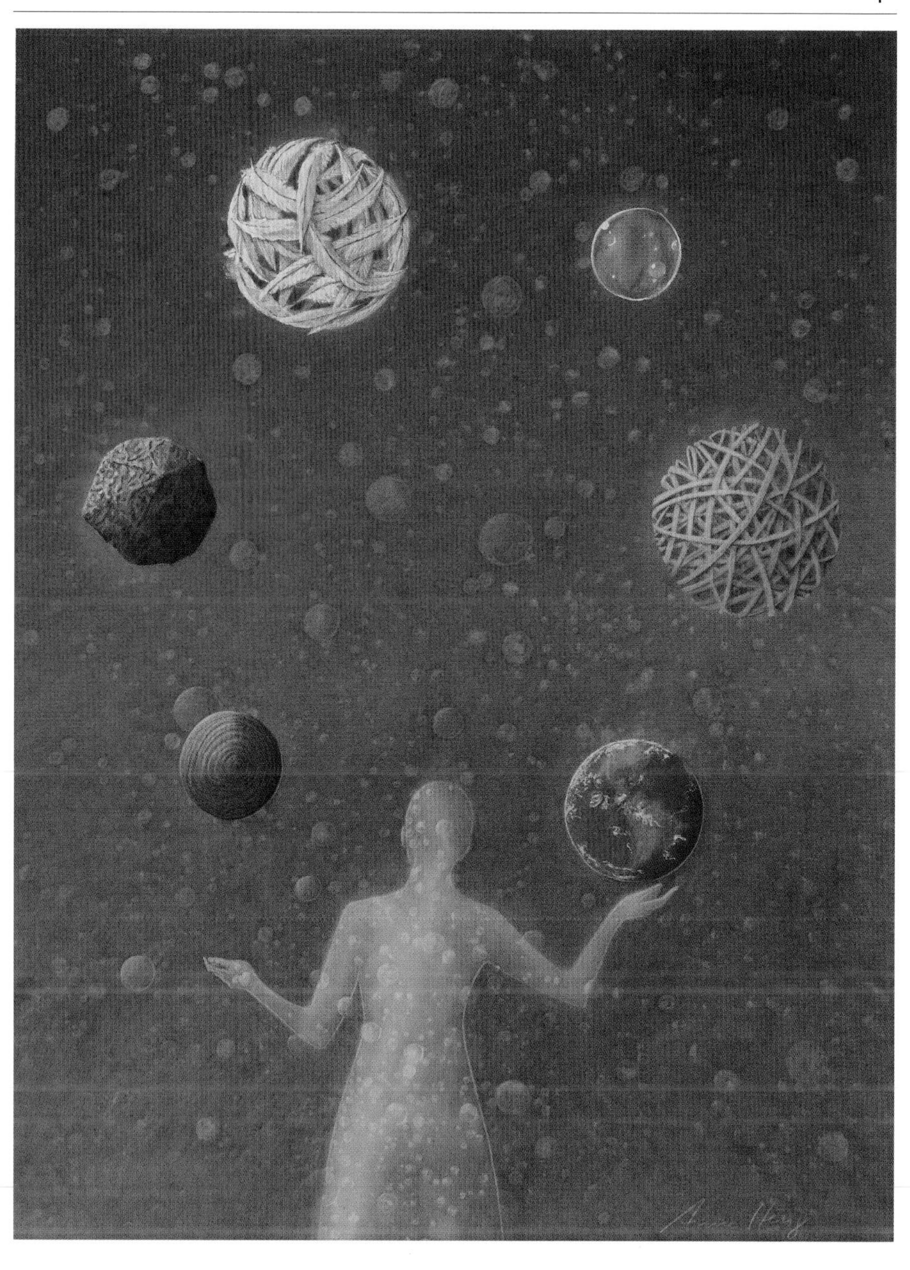

# Heart

Placed in the flow of life, my rhythm and my warming gush powerfully direct the fabric of body and soul into the most distant corners. With sensitivity I register even the smallest impulses and synchronize the interplay of organs as far as and including the spiritual levels.

This is my territory, in which I protect with all my strength all that is connected with me. Through the rhythm of tension and relaxation my innermost impulses are carried into the world like ripples in a pond, and my soul chambers receive the boundlessly diverse resonances of the universe.

Whether stone, plant, animal or human being, I am connected with the core of existence and know the deep feeling of belonging with all that is living. In this form of love, out of the innermost emerges an active compassion in which even unpleasant truths do not hurt.

My comprehensive wisdom dispels unclarity and imparts necessary answers from the realms of the feeling soul that follow a deep inner understanding. This opens new gates for love and creates room for undreamt-of realities to come into a person's life.

This applies in particular to the dialogue between two hearts, where my rhythm accompanies love in its mighty flow. Ensouled with this force of life, two human beings can change the course of the world.

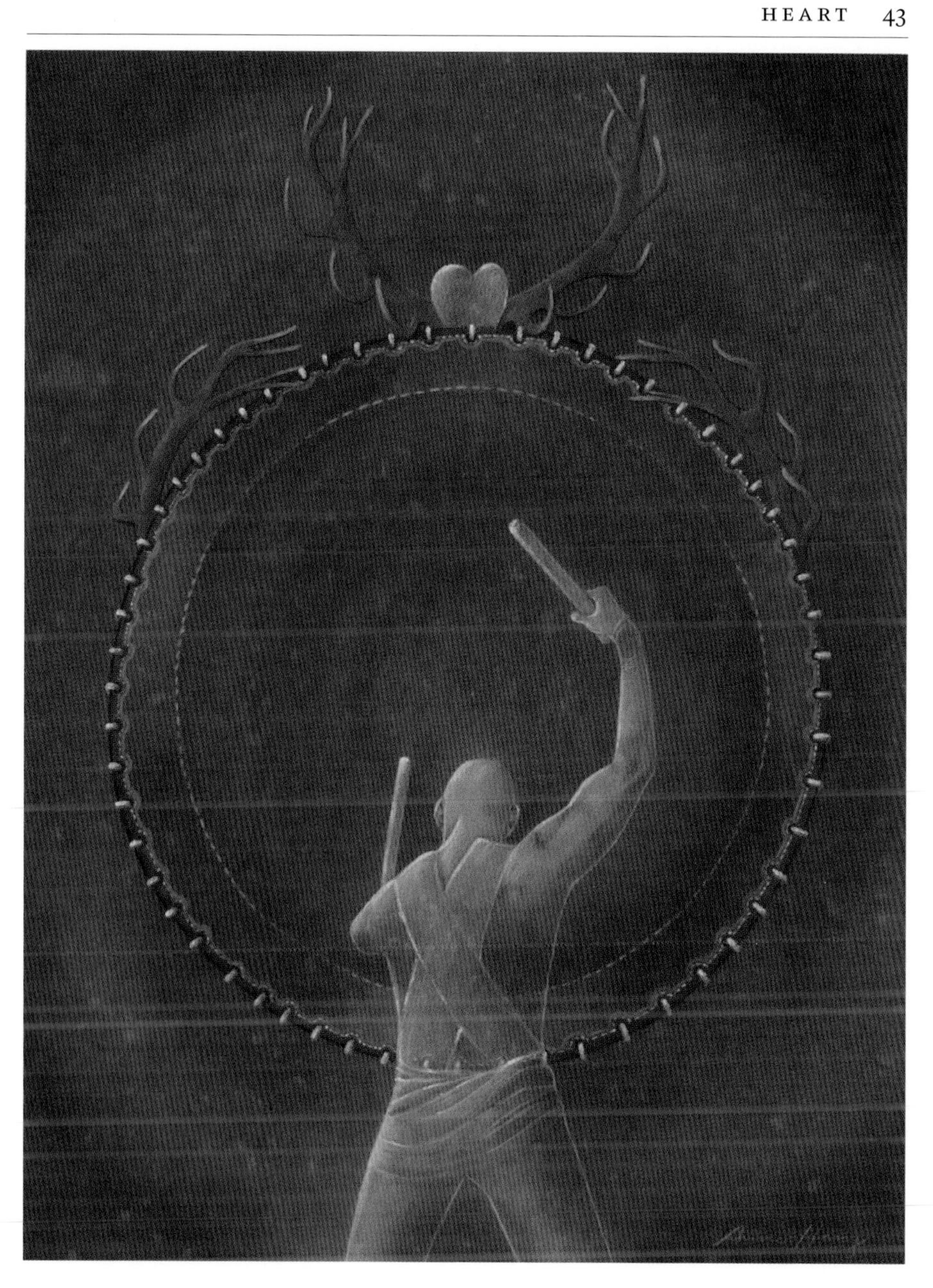

# Hip

If we talk about realizing goals or intentions I am the generator who makes the energies for this available. The middle point between my left and my right sides marks hereby the inner centre point of the person, his or her centre of mobility. From here I direct the dance of muscles and joints, here each wave of the breath discharges, and from here I start the prime movers in order to reach our goals in versatile determination. Whatever obstacles are in the way, my basic impulse is: "This also can be overcome!"

Jointly with the pelvic structure I form the sexual arc of tension. Here I operate in a fine inconspicuous vibration as well as with powerfully spreading pelvic movements as the mainspring for man's evolution.

I am the linchpin of the human erect posture and the basis of inner balance. Because of this, movements originating at my centre have a far-reaching effect. They not only allow us to reach a desired destination but can also promote ideas and carry them like torches into the world.

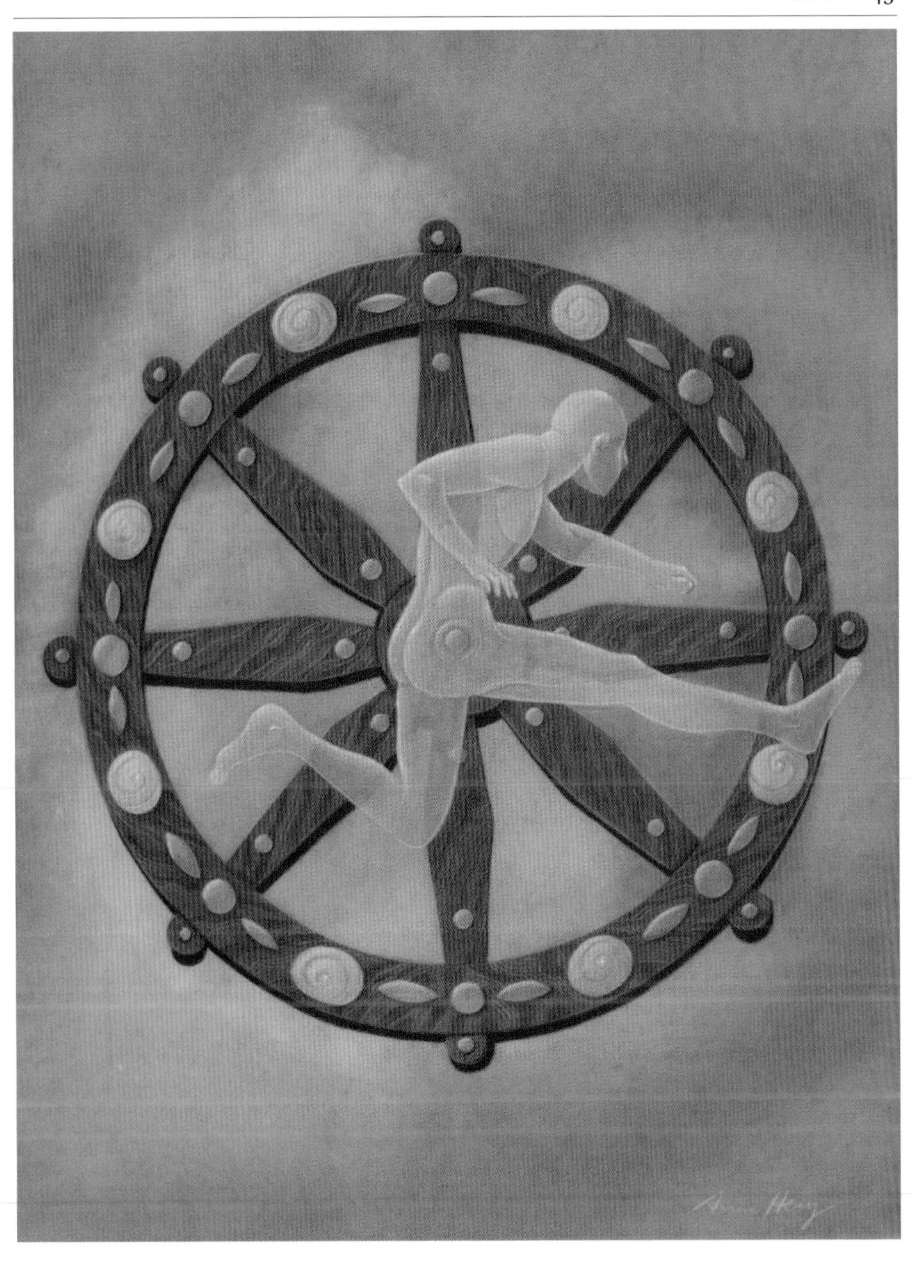

# Intestine, large

My task consists in concentrating on the essential. This includes the physical aspects, the handling of emotions and, in a much wider sense, everything that has to do with the topics of value and possession.

With my strength I focus energies, condense all material matter and enable basic values to radiate in full brilliance. Whether in the final phase of digestion or in the less visible aspects of the spiritual realm, I reduce everything to what is truly important.

This also applies to thoughts, feelings and energetic impulses. I retrieve the useful out of the available and simply let go of the rest. With the rhythm of focusing, accepting and letting go I provide a calm competence, an inner wealth that is fed out of the security of abundance.

Thereby I accept that values shift. When I attach great importance to something today, I recognize that tomorrow it may be significant in a different way. This awareness nourishes a zest for the abundance of life, for a willingness to enjoy everything and be satisfied with the best.

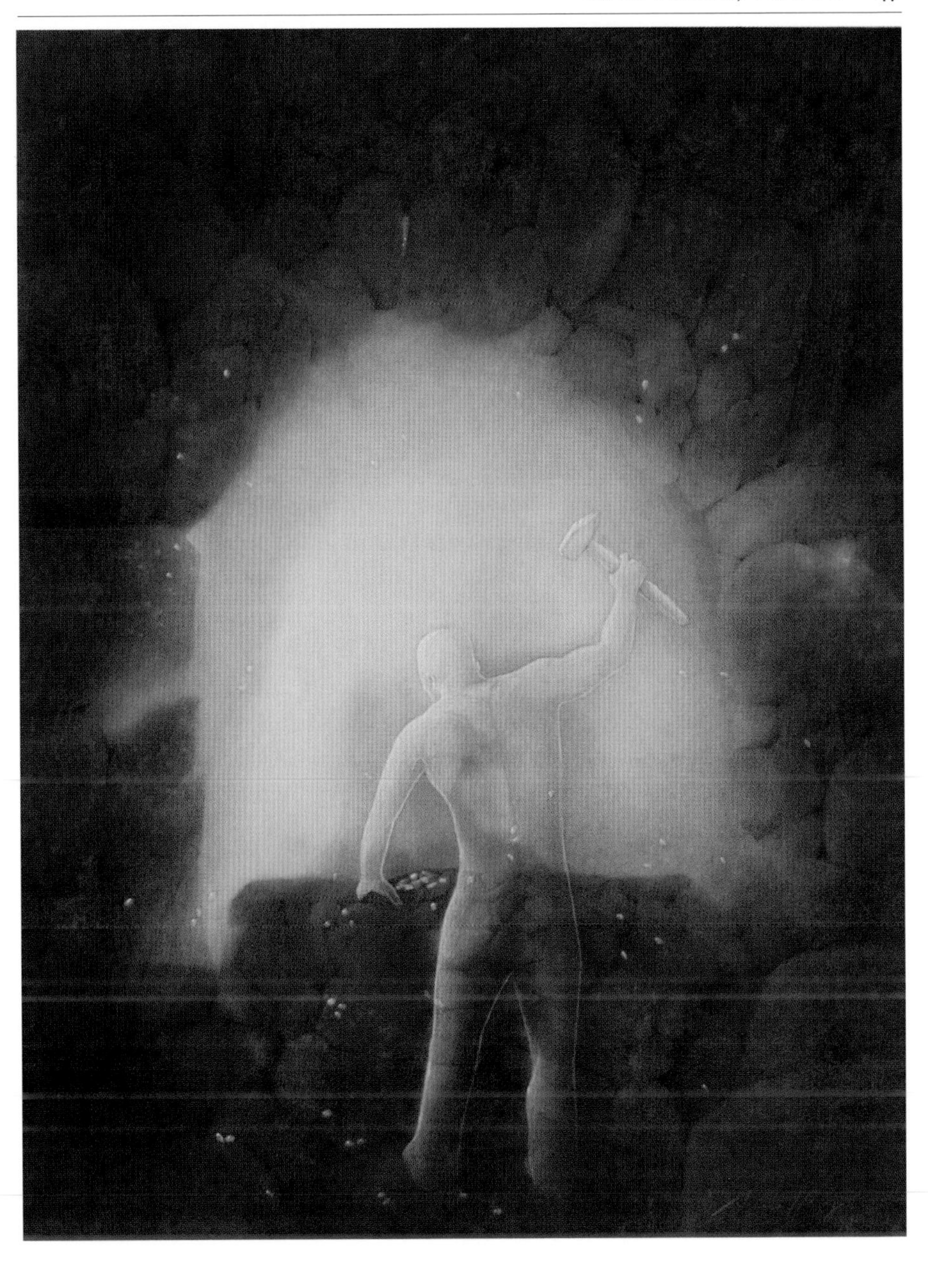

# Intestine, small

I am the guardian of my self-created big web. I retrieve the beneficial elements of food and guide the gratuitous through. In order to do so I have, from very early on in a person's life, woven a huge web around the intestines, which is closely linked to the emotions. Ever since then, thoughts and notions trigger an immediate "gut feeling". In addition, I guard and give background support to the immune system.

Everyone knows my language: a gush in the abdomen, full of relish, attests to comfortable circumstances. On the other hand we can count on conflicts and strain to come when decisions are accompanied by a queasy feeling.

My signals from the belly thus signify sympathy as well as dangers. Thereby I offer the individual reliable clues to the vital questions: What serves life and what could harm us. Thus in my web I pay particular attention to the threads that are connected with affection, security and self-worth.

By weaving these threads together I can successfully transform aversions, threats and anxieties and remove the rest from my web. Throughout this life-long process I form a stable personality that can enjoy beauty and is also equipped to deal successfully with problems.

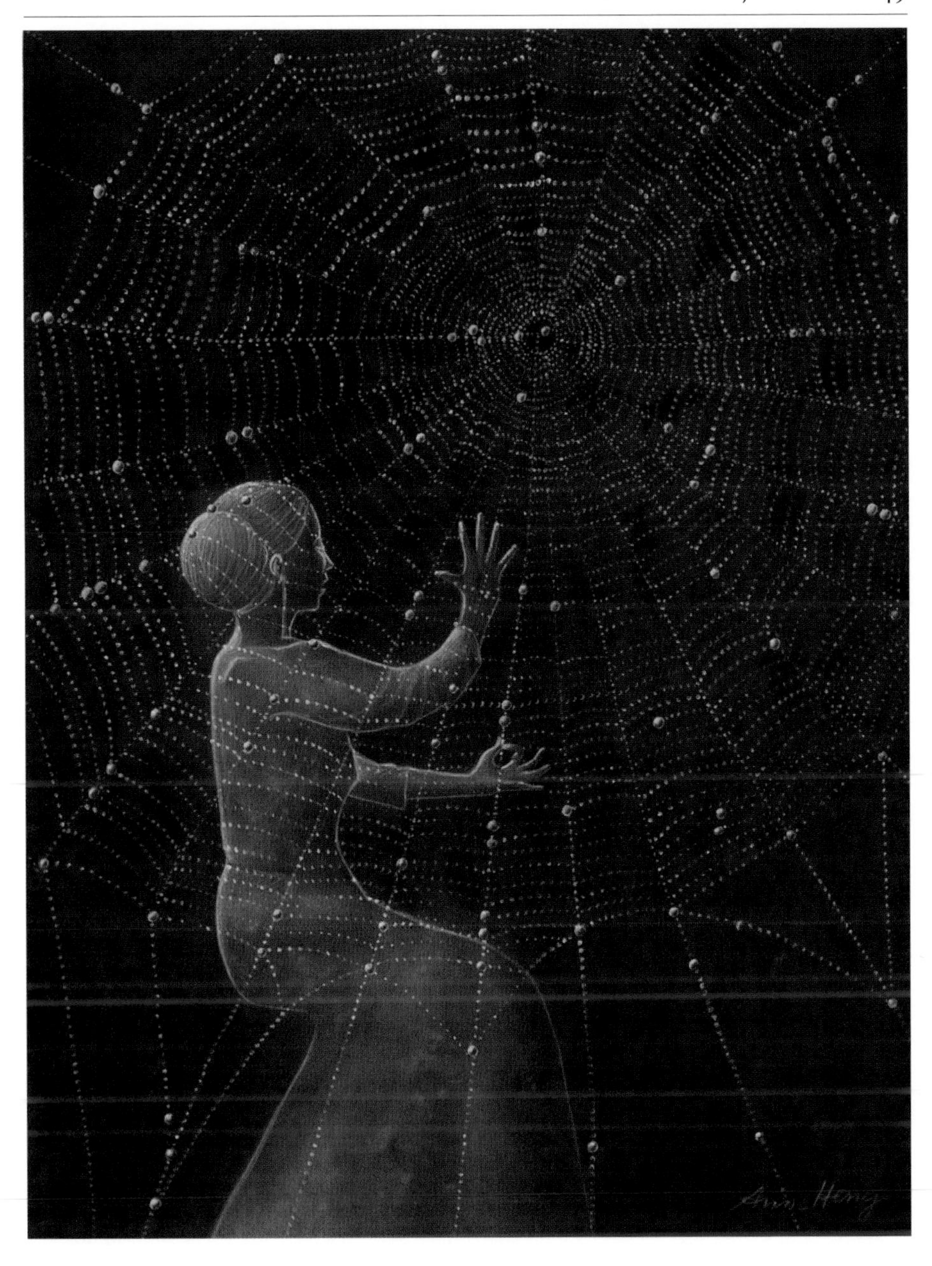

# Kidneys

We are life-giving and the source of stability of a highly alive soul animus, born of water and light. Concentrating the light of consciousness, we light the essence of the free will and allow the emotions' soul rivers to flow in emotional clarity.

"Do what you want", that is our motto. This implies doing what life commands out of its inner core. This means to intervene in the necessities of life via an active non-acting, and to transform the obstacles of life through loving compassion by turning towards them.

Like flowing water we can increase the energy for this, level upon level, until love takes effect in its purest form. For these tasks we are connected with the ocean of the ancestors. Their collected streams of thoughts and emotions, from the beginning of time, contain the sense of basic trust and the inspirations of the universe. With these deep unconscious soul aspects we open the gates of choice and guarantee that we always choose the best possible option – with the insight that this can change to another one a moment later.

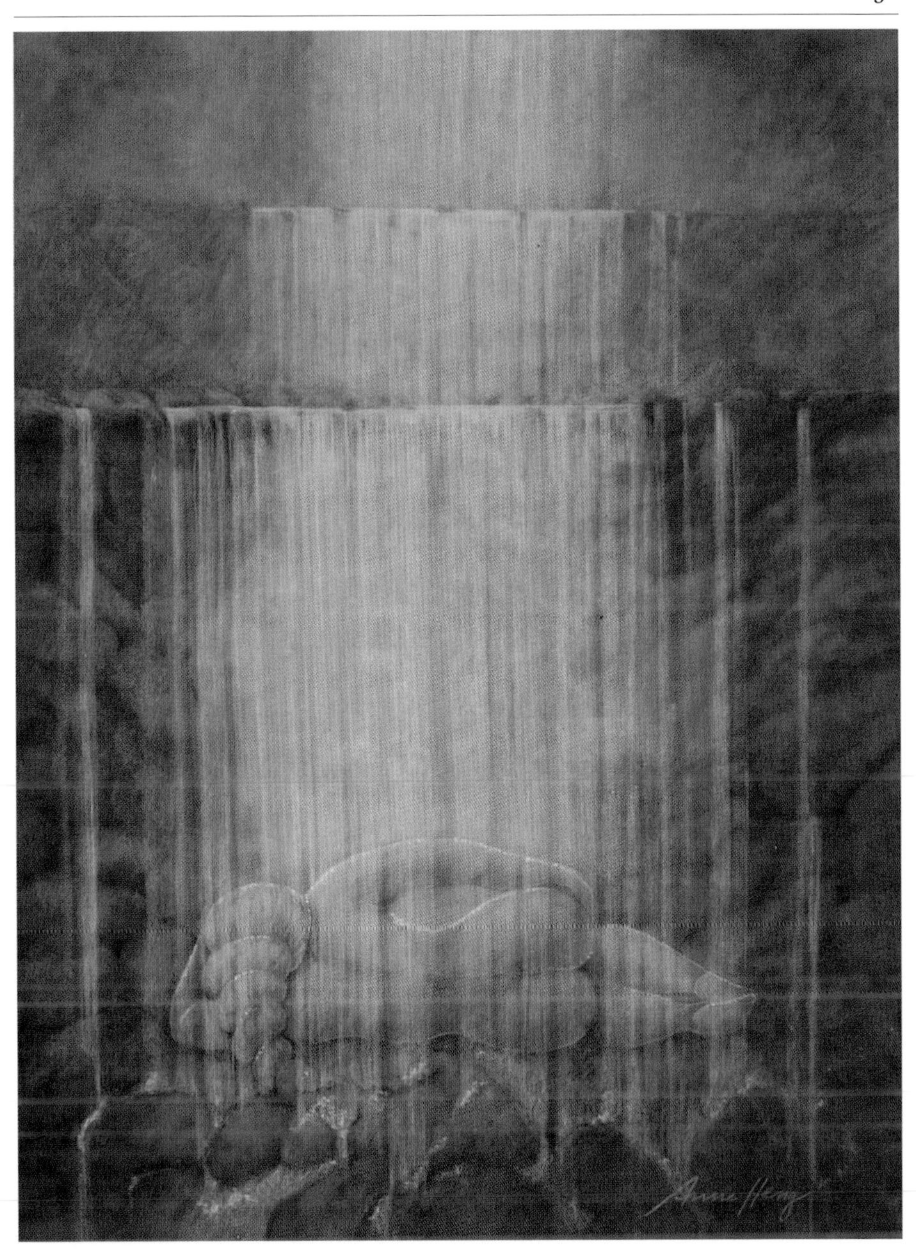

# Knees

We form the centre for the passage of the earth forces into the body and, with relish, unite the whole being with the dance of life. Through this we guarantee a stable flexibility in the earthly gravity field, where we ourselves then provide a safe equilibrium and stability even when the foundations start to wobble.

Via our resilient elasticity we control the rising energies in the spine, bring elegance to the body's posture and give emphasis to the implementation of all matters. This can be tangible, in particular when our epiphyseal cartilage closes, signifying the last step into adulthood.

In the interplay between bending and stretching we disclose the dignity of existence: In stretching we unfold a realization of life, in which the importance in life becomes perceptible, and in bending we serve the universe in loving dedication to it of all our strength. Through this rhythm we win our place in the fabric of the world as well as the safe trust that in each encounter we are equal.

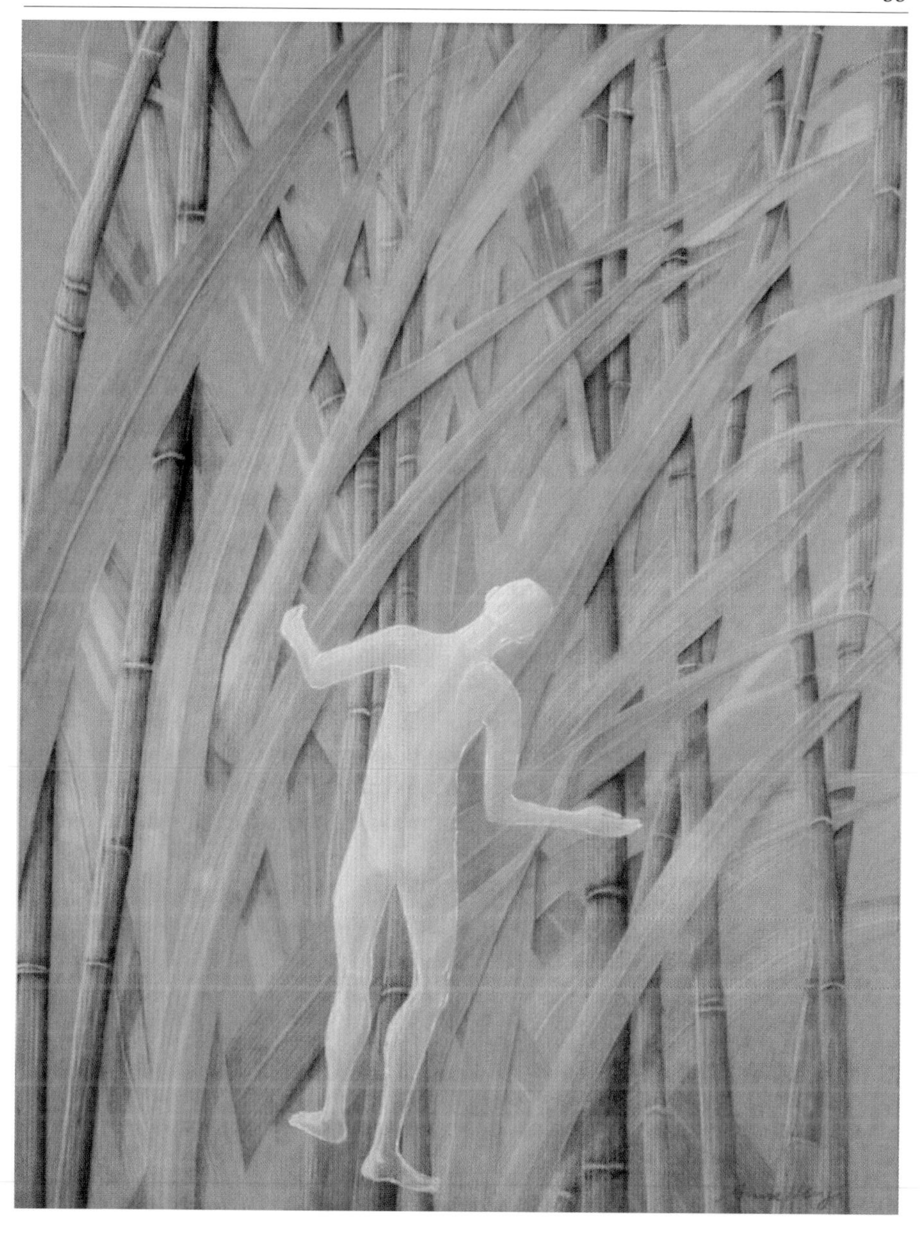

## Liver

I am the central organ of metabolism for body and soul. Whether nutrients, emotions or thoughts, through my way of operating I appropriate the environment for us.

To do this I transform the absorbed nourishment into fuels and building materials, modify them and, if necessary, detoxify them. In equal measure I examine mental and spiritual impulses, situations and encounters with regard to their coherence.

In connection with my ability to develop strategies I provide a stable sense of self-worth for the human being. Thus I can make use of the abundance of life, store energies and remove superfluous remains from body and soul.

Connected with this is my task of always providing the person with the optimal amplitude of energy. This also encompasses our liquid life force, the blood. I am of particular service to this elixir; I keep it within its boundaries and maintain its flow.

With all these skills I give the person access to their powers of self-determination in order to be happy. Thus, ultimately, I am the authority for a laughing creativity that channels pathways from the innermost, so that life and love may succeed.

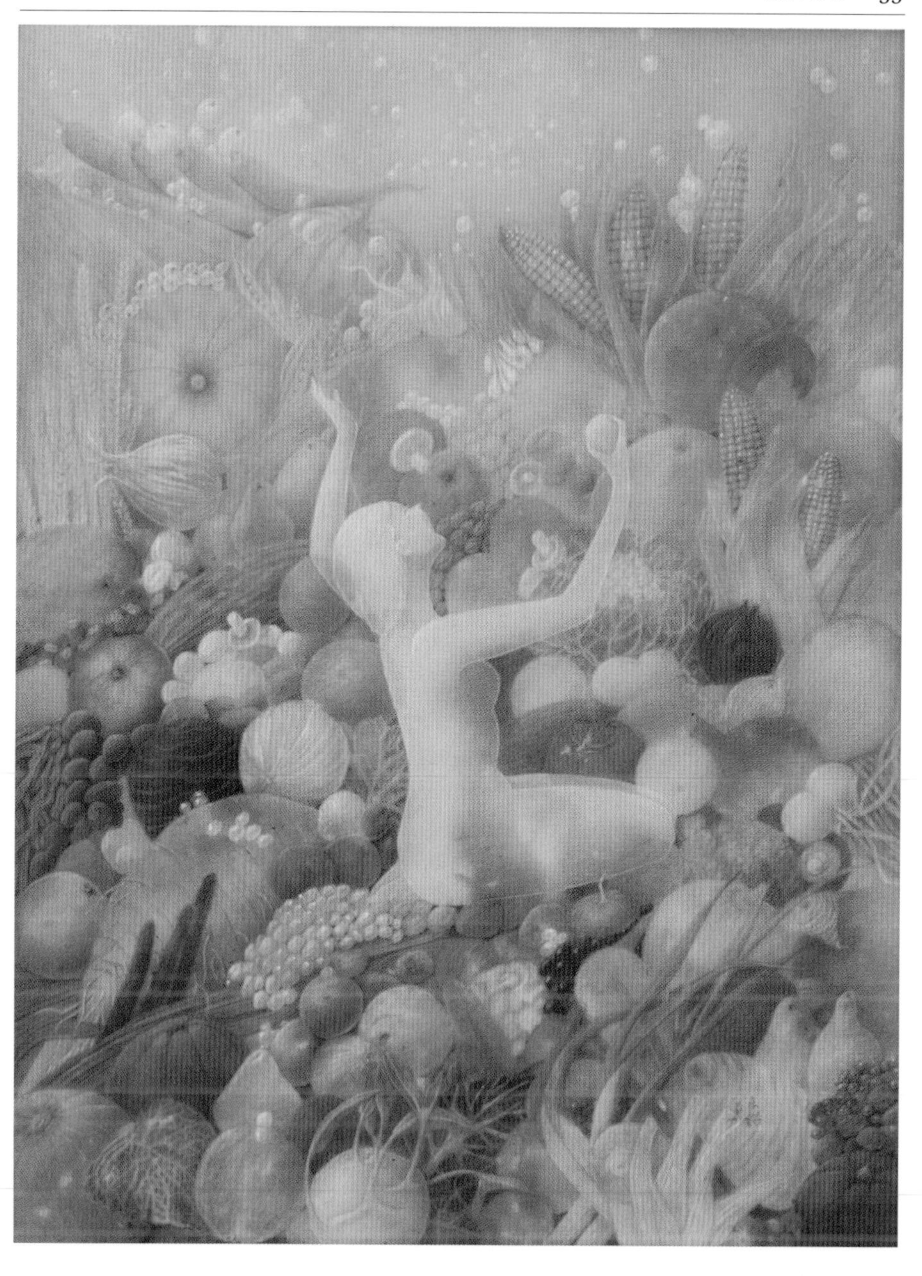

# Lungs

From the first cry to the last breath my powerful wings follow the rhythm of life. My force has many names: Prana, breath or chi. They are all an expression for the current of life energy that arises out of the inner self.

This energy flow disperses in endless form through body and soul, in order to start anew with the next breath following its reunion with its source. At the cusps of these movements we connect the interior with the exterior world. These are exactly the moments in which we reveal the mystery of coming into existence and passing from it, this is where we bring the pulse of the universe into life and keep endowing the pendulum between self-preservation and surrender with a new impulse.

In this cycle we are at home in all elements. Our breath, like fire, can kindle all life on a spiritual level, the waters of our soul can lead to the sheer fathomless depths of the emotions; our earth cave conveys a safe feeling of security and our breezy wings soar towards a clear overview.

In the mindful balance of heart and reason our strengths find their expression in the word. This allows our energies to be directed everywhere, including to the organs; though these have already known us anyway, for since the beginning of time they have been swaying languorously in the rhythm of our wings.

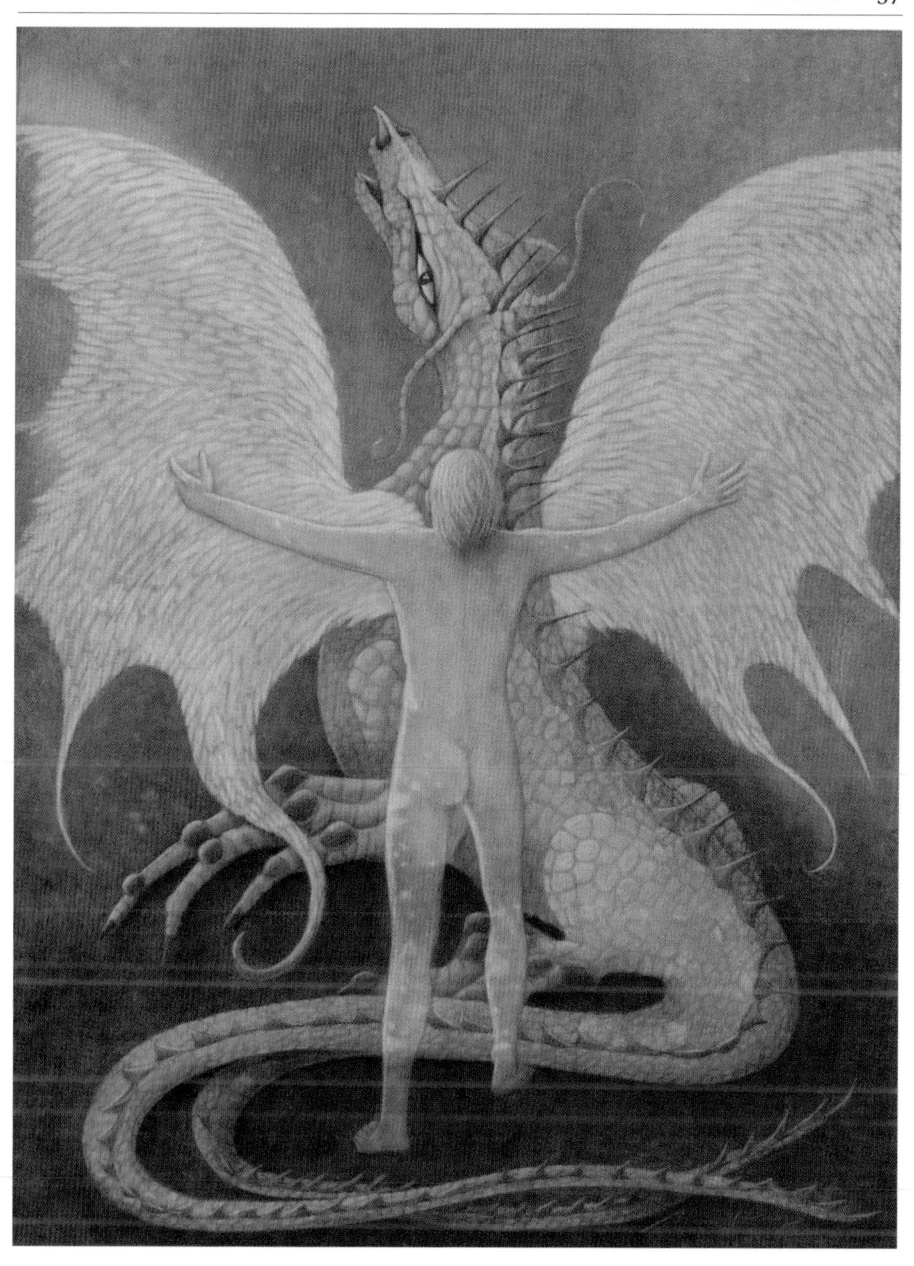

## Mammary Gland

Even though birthing as a form of mothering is reserved for women I also embody the nourishing sensitivity in men. I am the source of security, care and belonging that is significant for everything emerging anew.

Whether newborn children or ideas, conceived from the universe they come into the world after an inner process of maturing and, with the help of the female nesting energy, need to be helped gently over the hurdles of their initial tender phase until they are strong enough to exist in the world.

In all beginnings lives the enchantment of the new. I nourish this impulse with my love and care for its growth with dedication. Thereby I accompany developments and make people happy, which allows them to experience their significance in life. I reveal that all that emerges is a snapshot of perfection. Herein becomes visible the seed of an even more magnificent consciousness that after being born also continues to need my care.

Ultimately, I am thus one of the essential foundations of all growth and developments that accompany a stable feeling of self-worth.

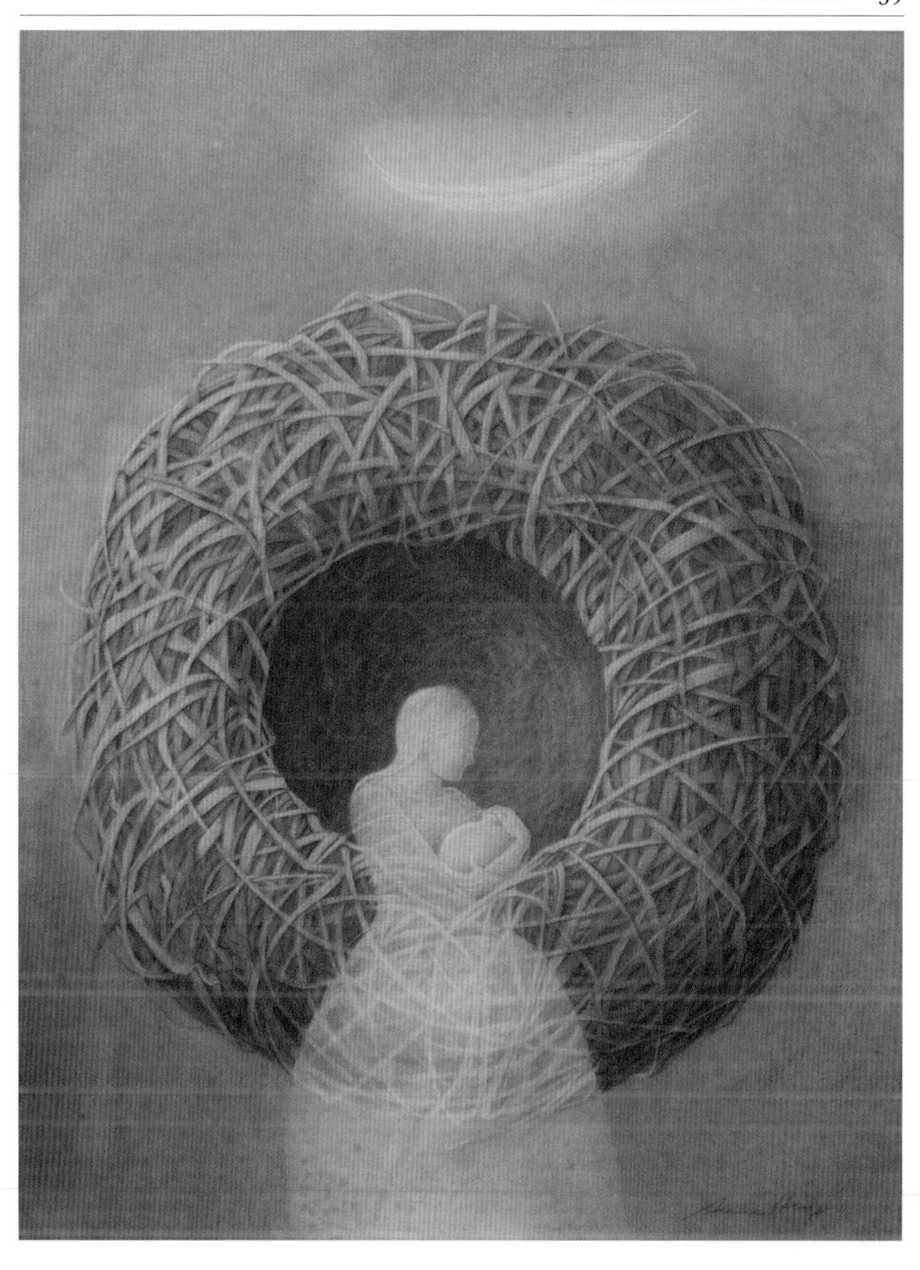

## Nose

As guardian of the sense of smell I possess skills far beyond that of the ability to scent.

Even the distinction between edible and inedible is not restricted to food alone but also extends to the people we meet and surround ourselves with. Here it becomes obvious that I am a powerful mentor for life as I direct the attention towards enjoyable as well as dangerous circumstances.

This applies in a much more refined and distinctly more profound way to sexuality. As we evaporate our own odour when we sweat, are excited and court a woman or a man, my scent-sensing antennae recognize instinctively who matches us at heart, who we are attracted to sexually, who leaves us unconcerned and who we just cannot stand.

This basic sense of trust in my perceptions is directed by my memory of smells that follow the deep emotions. This way my perceptions allow me to unmistakably pinpoint the leads to both opportunities and dangers.

With this, I catch the scent of where the twists of life take a wholesome turn. Not least among these are the ways to pleasure, joie de vivre and success.

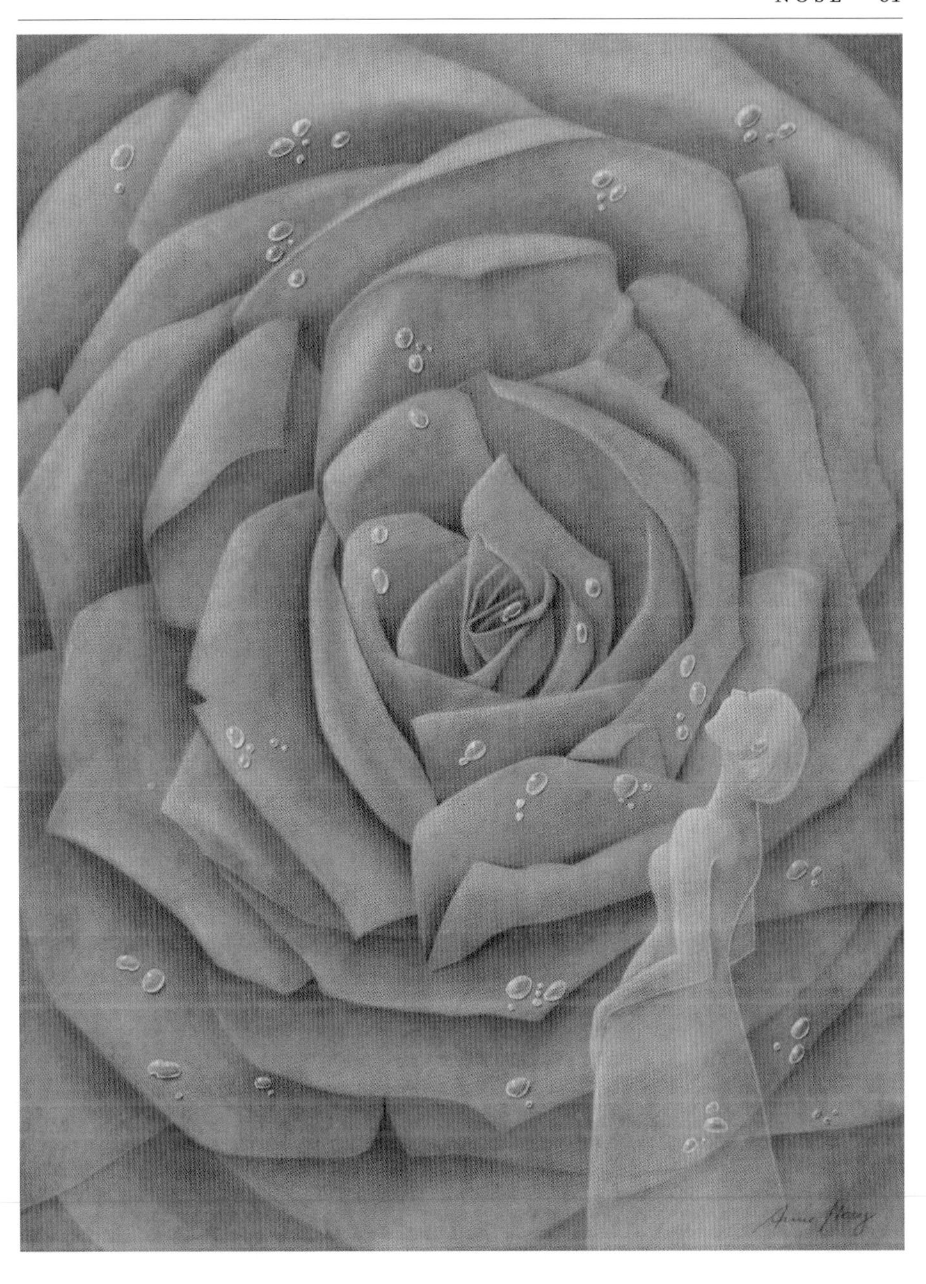

## Pancreas

Out of my cornucopia the stream of wish-fulfilment pours. I satisfy longings and provide all levels of the human being with nourishing experiences that find their goals in creative engagement and a healthy evolvement of the life force.

In my basic function I act as energy provider for body and soul. Physically my digestive enzymes and my hormones see to supplying the cells well with energy from food.

Equally important though are my tasks in the realm of mind and soul. As guardian of the cornucopia I give off the abundance of life. “Be generous” is my motto and with this I also claim it.

If I am perceived in this way there is always more than enough. Then I can transform all wishes and longings to gratitude and operational energy, as all the richness of this world is always at our disposal.

Thus through me pleasures find their climax, but also their transformation into soul impulses. Following the path of ecstasy encourages undreamt-of energies to start to flow so they can then find their place in life as lived insights.

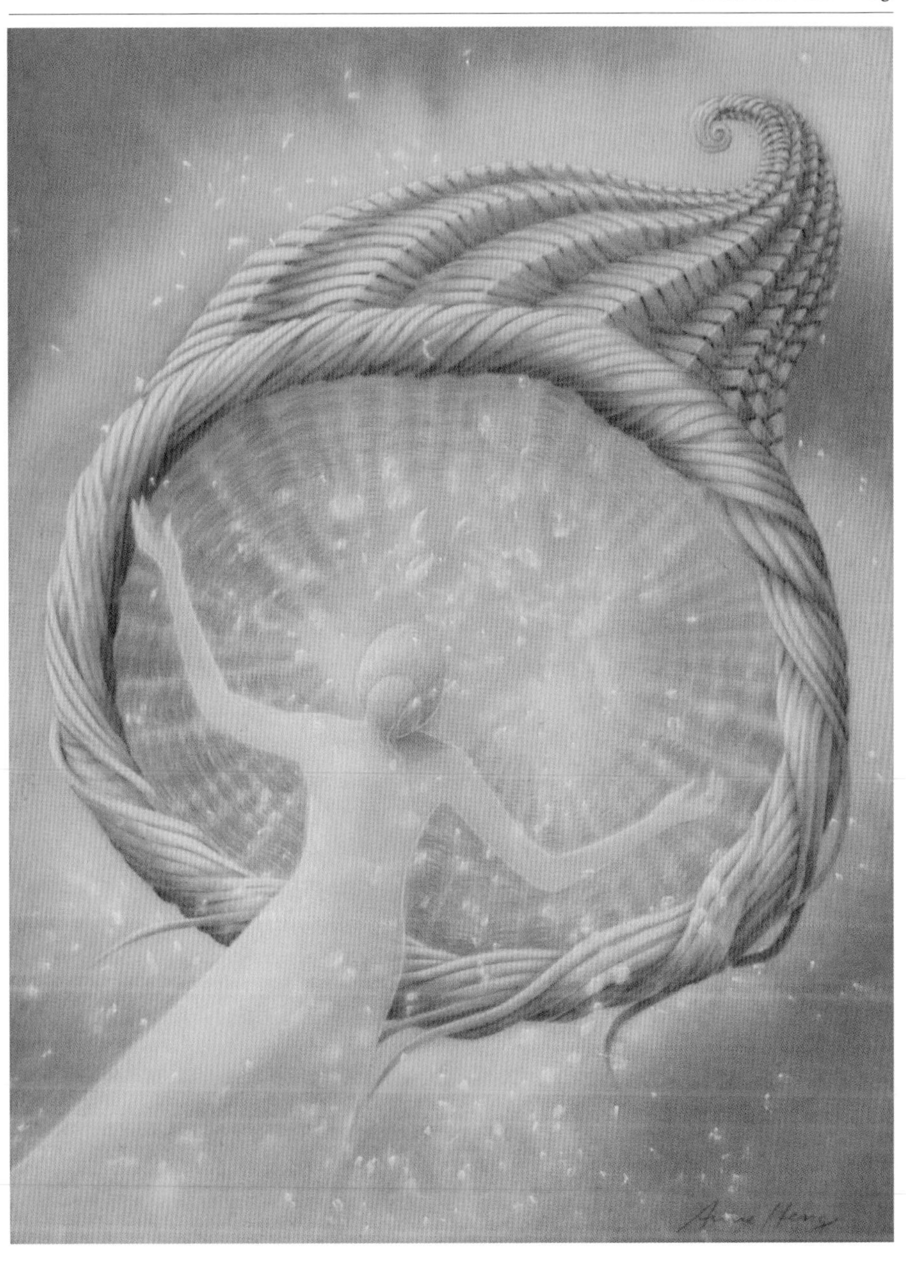

# Reproductive Organs, female: Uterus, Ovaries and Vagina

Initially, we make ourselves known only very quietly and convey sensations that comprise the whole body as languorous shivers. These are the signals of the female sexuality, the creative basic power of the Eros, that want to be awakened from the heart.

This tender blossom we nourish in puberty with an increasing confidence in the sense of being a woman, so that she can grow to discover the appetite in these life impulses and to experience erotic desire.

Our hormones build the body for this and open the portals to the ocean of being a woman, where the female identity is at home with her most unique rhythms, which pulsate in accordance with the tides of the world.

With this female moon pulse we are the creative force of life itself that follows a clear rhythm: We open the woman for acting in the world, and in return we regenerate the forces in the waters of the earth.

In such self-determination we can promote the pleasure of the sexual energy exchange and serve the man as mirror for his hidden female elementary forces.

Our task consists in expressing the receiving principle, growing with pleasure and opening the inner woman for a devoted love, also in order to birth new life in the treasure chamber of evolution.

To recognize a man then means to meet him in the depth of the soul and in the union celebrating existence.

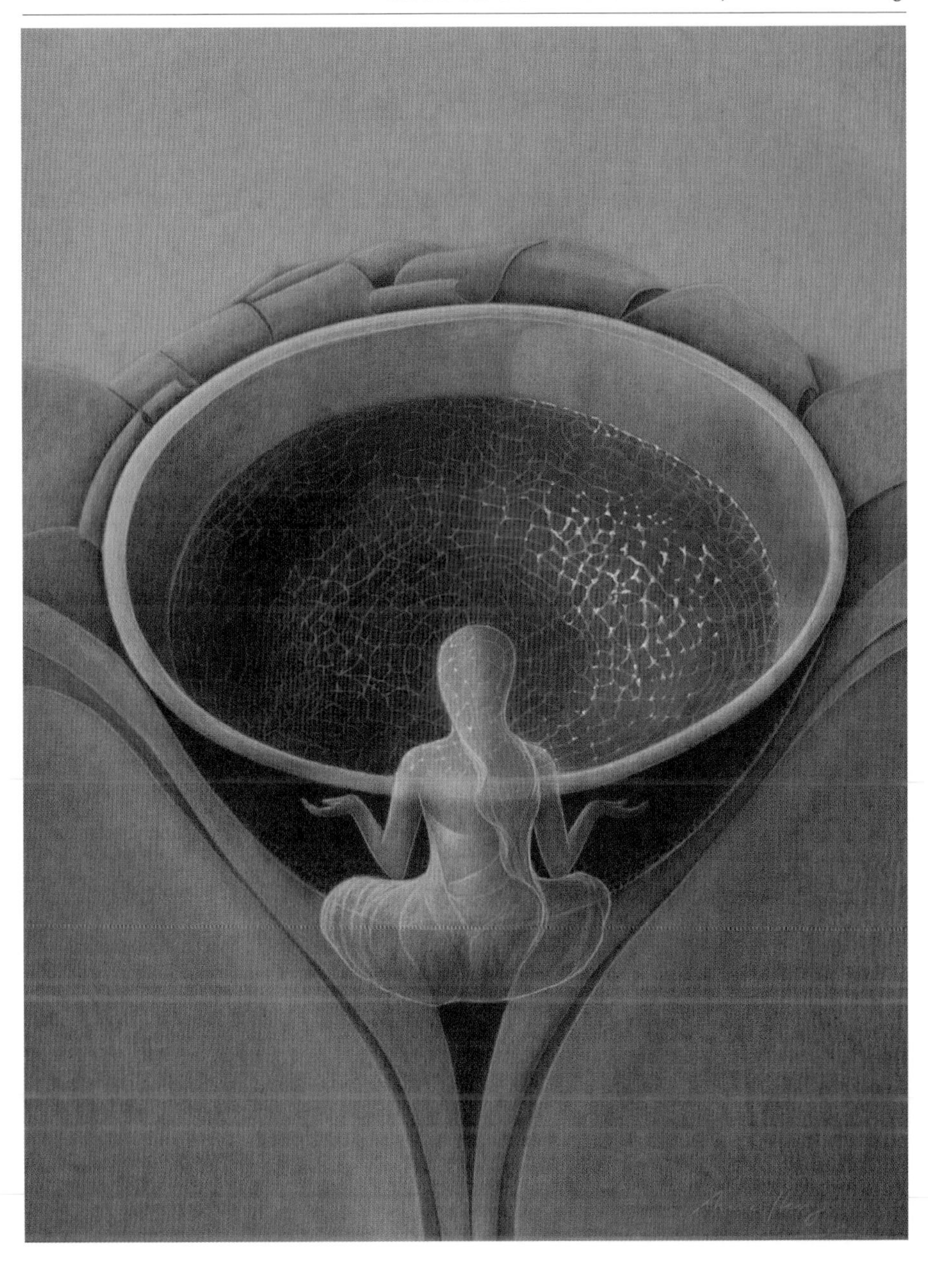

## Reproductive Organs, male: Penis, Testicles, Prostate Gland

When we delight a boy for the first time with a pleasurable ejaculation he is mostly confused. Here we blend a never-before-experienced sensation of desire carrying a sweet inner melting with a deeply felt awakening. With this experience we clear the path to growing up.

We are the guardians of the male sexuality, the creative base force of the Eros, that want to be awakened from the heart. Through the male hormones we open the man up for the beauty of the feminine.

Hereby we unfold the urge in him to give his semen to life, to move the world and to unfold an aggressive creativity. The rise of the lingam, the sceptre of lust, is a symbol that opens the man up to the fascination of experiencing the depths of the feminine with consciousness and of serving the woman as mirror for her hidden masculine elementary power.

This involves the opportunity to grow in a dedicated sexual love and to develop a healthy self-confidence in which even insecurity can be a form of strength.

Recognizing a woman thus means allowing being touched beyond touch in order to encounter the essence of the woman in the depth of the soul.

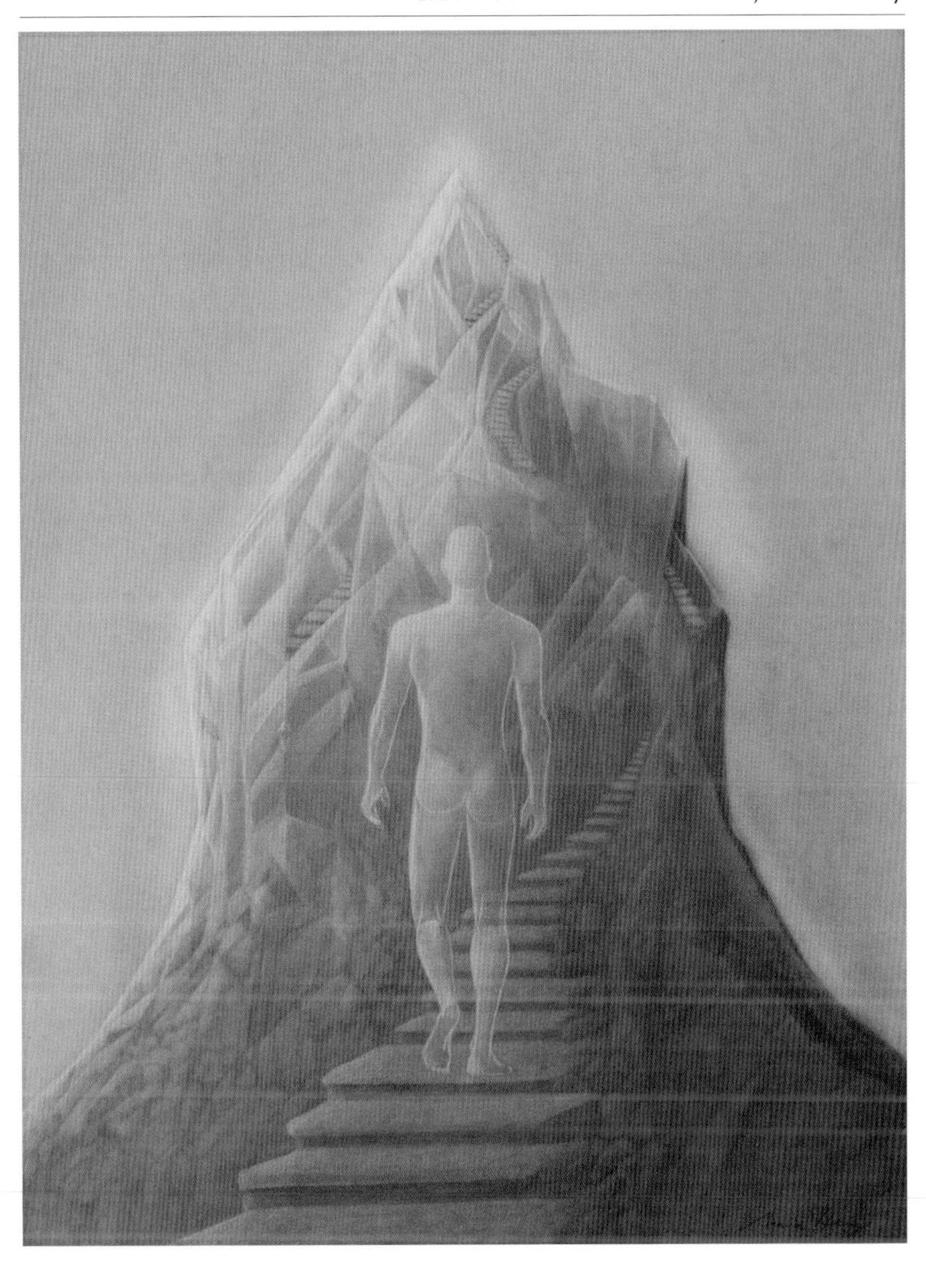

# Shoulders

On me the world rests, and out of my centre I comprehend time and space, as dimensions, in their immeasurableness. In me is the space in which past and future are embedded in the infinity of the Now. Through my being I reveal ways that lead to the closeness of heartfelt embraces as well as securing self-preservation through vital boundaries.

If I invite the universe into my movement radius I communicate its powers to the inner. There they can be perceived as self-esteem and aligned attitude. In return, I open – through surrender – the inner spaces of the world's soul.

The dialogue of these two movements is the beat of the wing of a mighty angel that brings us into contact with our strength.

Moreover, we rediscover again and again the point of Archimedes in us, from where we can lift the world off its hinges. Trusting higher guidance, I assure the individual that the universe is whole, that we are a part of it and that we are granted the experience of this serendipity.

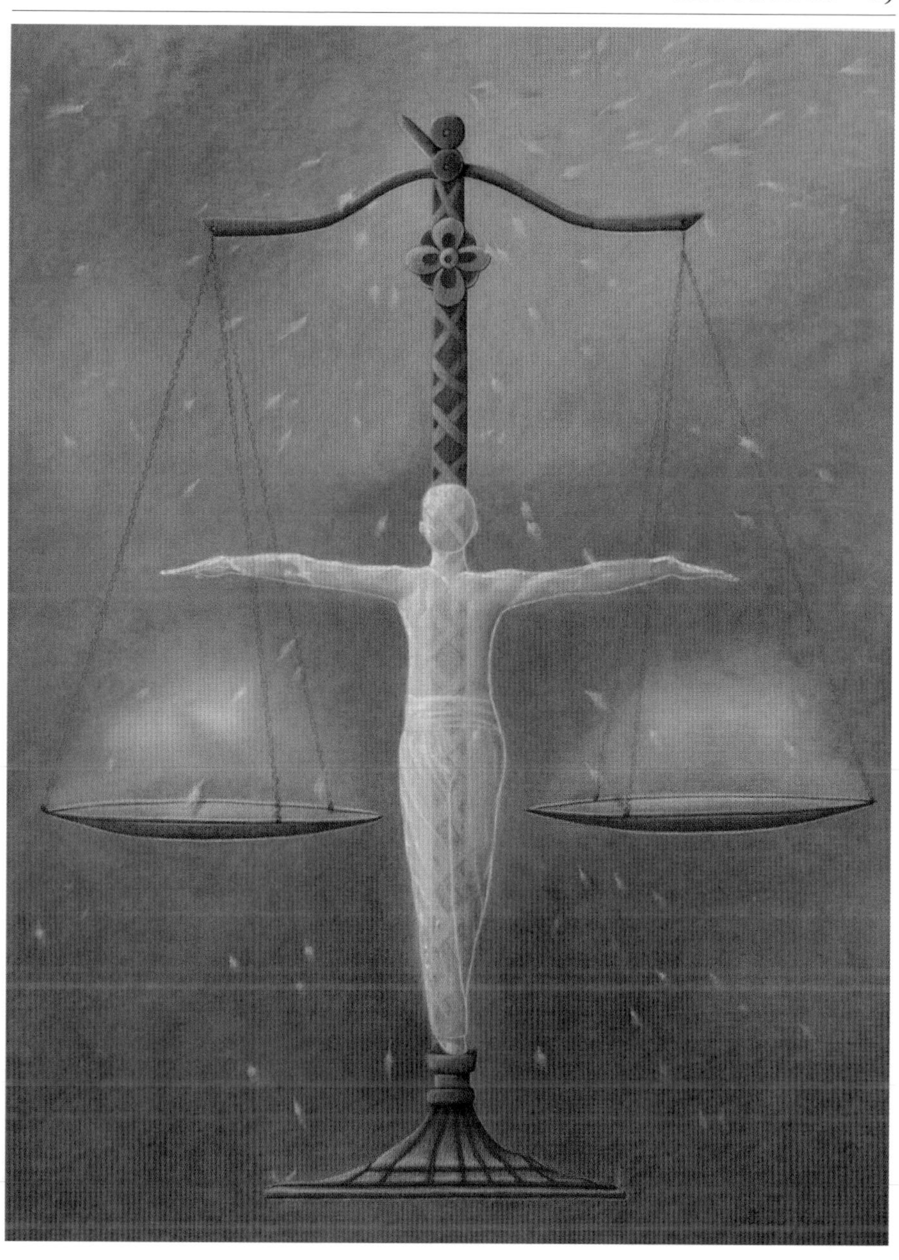

# Skin

I am the treasure of security, comfort and belonging, and I provide experiences that get us directly in touch with the core, while on the outside goose bumps form, feelings are gripped by a shiver, and sometimes even the floodgates of tears open with emotion.

Through this I enable a living exchange and vital contacts for the connection with the inner and from the inner to the outer.

At the threshold of the body we as humans receive assurance that everything inside of it belongs to us, and that therefore the outer world has to be something else. With this we gain self-awareness in the truest sense of the word.

In the course of life, I allow the human being through such borderline experiences to increasingly discover more of his or her self. I also convey the insight that the self does not end at the boundary of the body at all but comprises the entire field of the energy presence.

I maintain stable protection of the physical and energetic field that envelopes us. I bring into awareness the senses of closeness and distance, and open the energy field for friends and loving embraces.

This enables the individual to increase the energy field of their presence further and further, and to perceive occurrences that take place far outside the known senses. Ultimately, this includes the experience that there are no boundaries and that any limitations exist within our belief system alone.

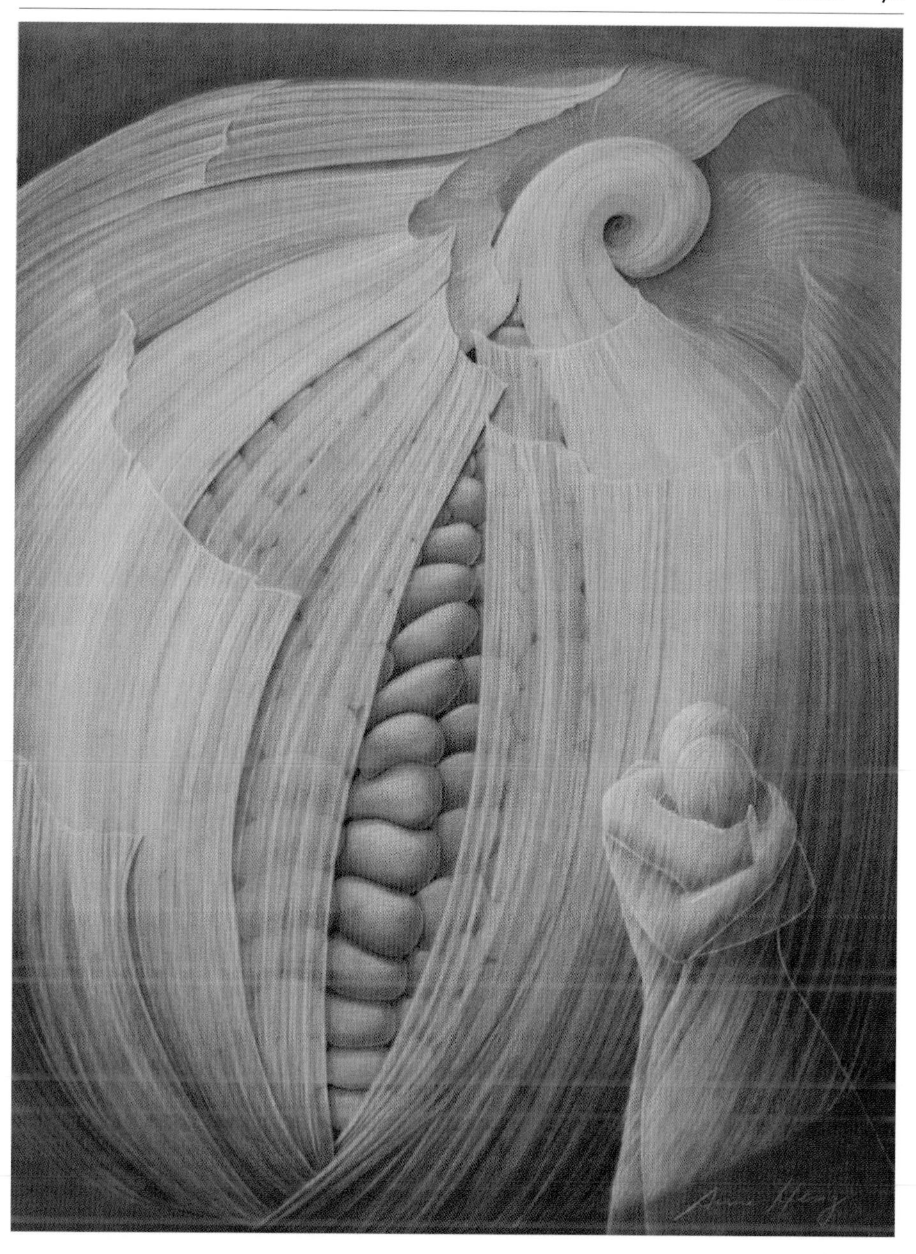

## Spine

Striving upwards while resting on strong roots, weathering the storms of life and flexibly following the course of the world; I am the Tree of Knowledge, the Tree of Life of the Kabbala or Yggdrasil, the World Tree of the Edda.

My basic theme is the same everywhere: "Find your own aligned position and meet the changes in life with flexibility."

With the energies that flow through me I guard a soul granary, which holds all experiences as attitudes, as know-how that props you up and as sincerity.

If the energy can flow freely through my granary I show this as a soft, nearly imperceptible caress through the back, as a flowing that comes forward in all colours and pitches of the emotions, or as sensations that move like blissful, almost insufferably beautiful showers through me.

In these moments, I connect the elementary world of earthbound matter with the spiritual planes of the divine spark.

Out of this comes a clear awareness of upcoming topics and the whole life journey; and since all organs and tissue are connected with me, these are also cared for and healed by this energy flow, as well as elevated in their energy levels.

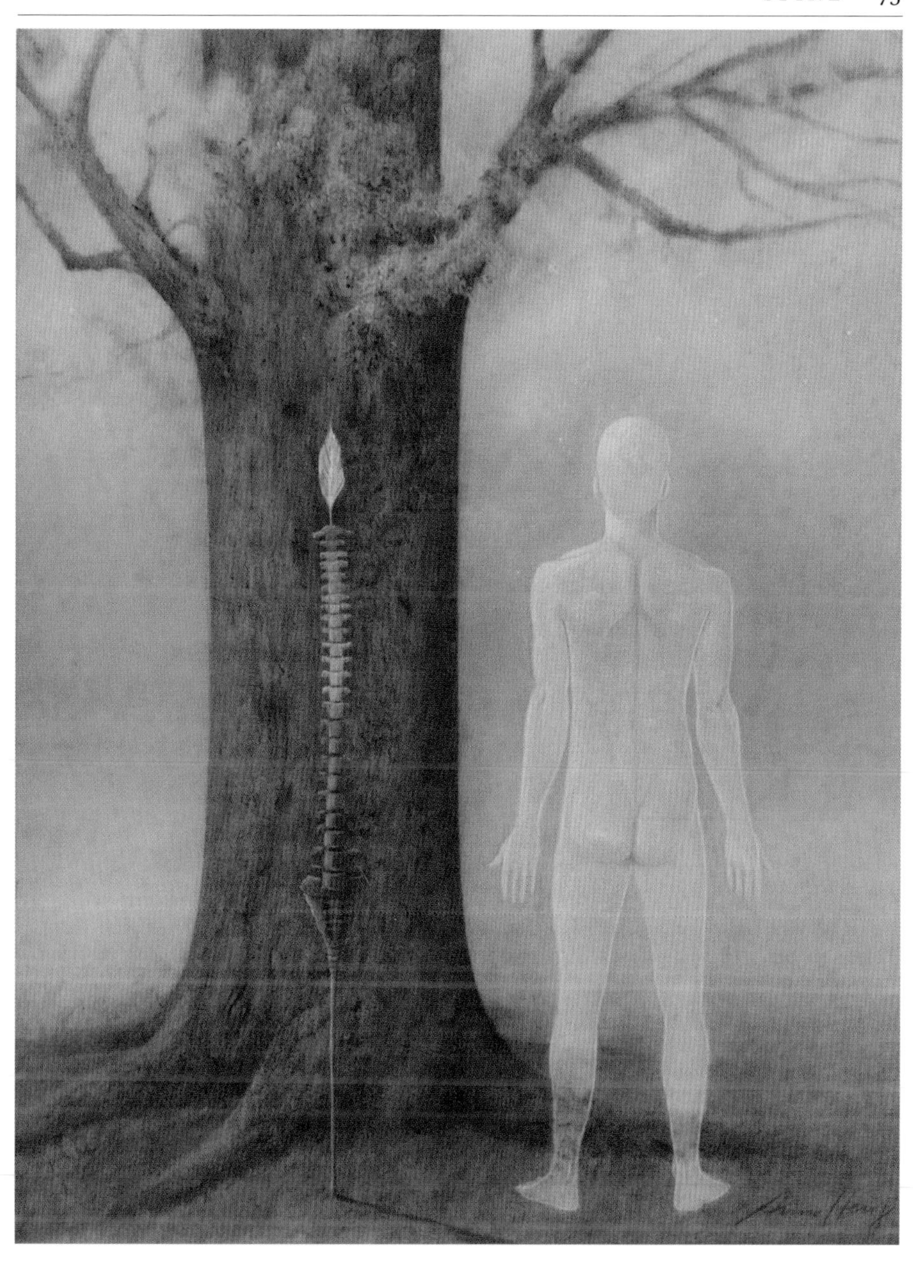

## Spleen

I am often misjudged, overlooked or even feared, even though I represent the assertion of independence of body and soul. The ancestors have even credited me with the significance of an inner sun that provides each individual cell with the rays of consciousness.

All these tasks I perform in mental clarity. Through sorting out old and worn-out blood cells, I guarantee good productive efficiency of the blood and thus of the individual. Furthermore, I train the elite defence units in my elite school, the immune system.

These physical aspects are the better known, although I stand for clarity on the soul level too. At the thresholds of the personality I guard the gateways to the stages of development.

In the transition from dependence during the baby phase towards the emotional self-expression of childhood, I control the floods of emotions that demand access at this point.

The next threshold is reached with the onset of the mind's activity. Here I am the guardian that arrests the thoughts that might overburden.

On the third threshold, in puberty, I stand at the transition towards coming of age. Here I fend off external influences in order to enable a positive development towards an independent personality while respecting the self. At this point, I am in particular charge of allowing the concepts of the previous generation to die, so that the human being in his/her continual rebirth can keep up with the evolution of the world soul.

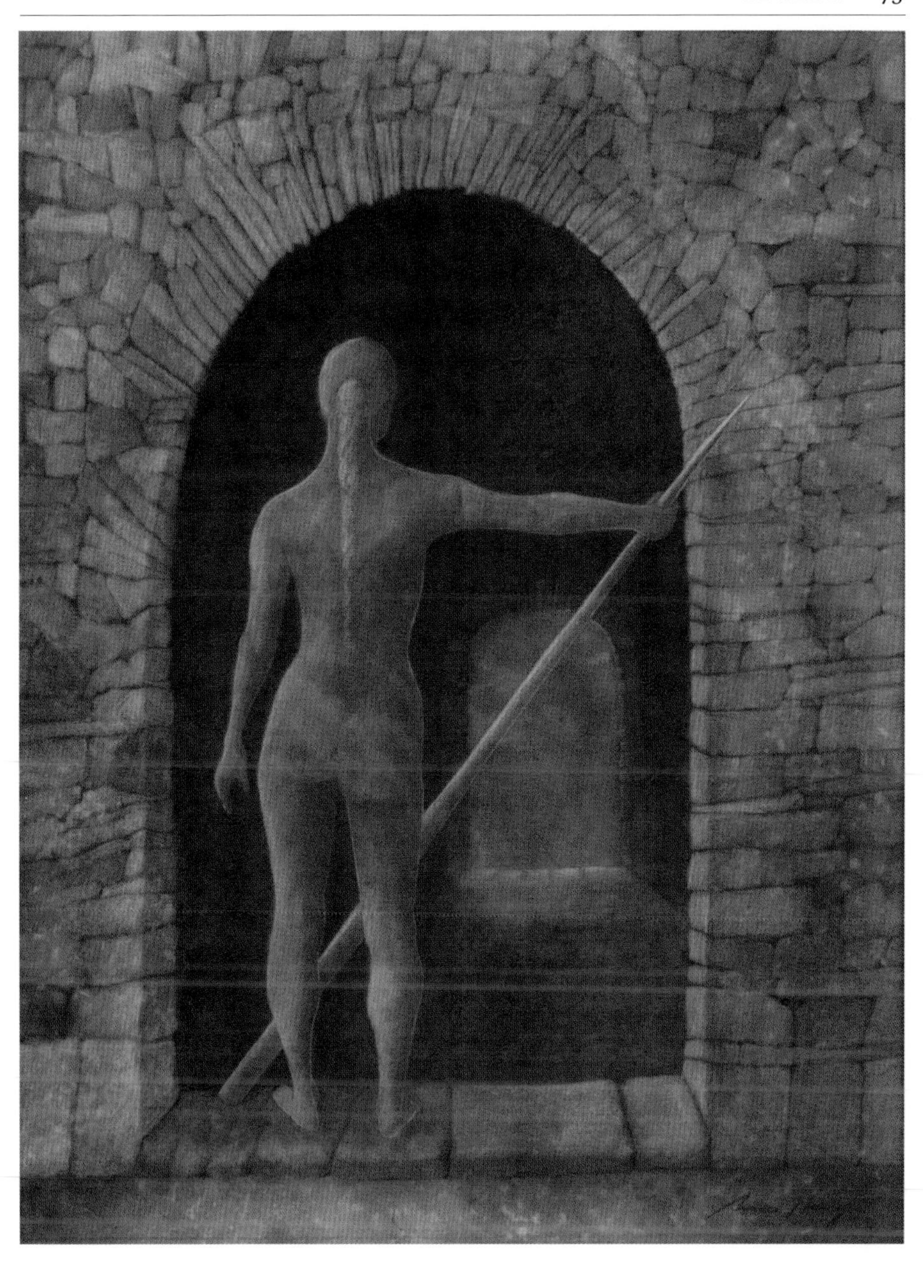

## Stomach

It is not only the food and drink with which my organ is filled that is being digested in my cauldron. I attend just as thoroughly to thoughts and emotions, as with these energies I nourish the soul.

All this I blend into a brew out of which arises the basic energy for life. The quality of the ingredients, the intensity of the inner fire and the mindfulness in handling my cauldron determine the harvest of energy that I can bring forth out of it.

Above all, natural foods and positive feelings let my cauldron naturally simmer with joy. When on top of that I receive benevolence, compassion and readiness for action my fire can blaze fully. From here I am in the position to transform all troubling influences – like ravenousness, cravings and conflicts – into insights.

With such a magic potion obsolete patterns are consumed by my flames, burdens vanish like smoke escaping and the deep human needs of acknowledgement gain a rebirth in love. Thus I transform heaviness and worries into a sense of well-being that is capable of acting.

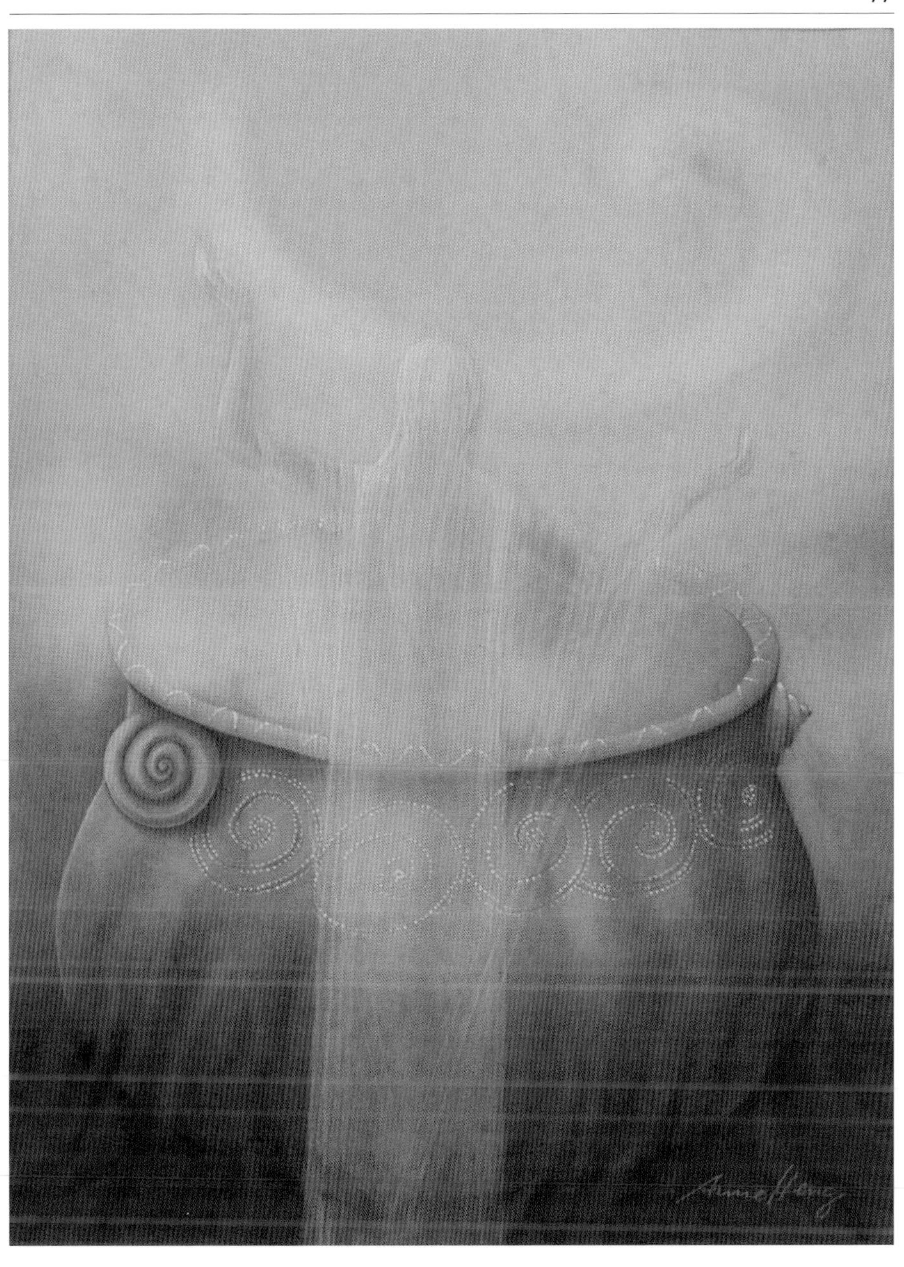

# Teeth

When it comes to primal instincts, we are the representatives that most explicitly bring to mind the joint heritage of all living beings and things.

With our ability to cut all food to small pieces and grind it we lend flexibility for producing energy. We form the hardest structure of the human being, that in the personality is expressed as willpower.

Indeed, a child's very set of us invites in the powers of will and assertion. Fed by the sources of an animalistic connection to nature and the consciousness fields of the ancestors, we thus stand for development into an independent human being who is ready to take his or her place in the world.

With the change of our first representatives to those of us that stay with you throughout life, we affirm each individual's justified claim to self-realization and its redemption in love. Connected to this is active alignment towards companions on the path to a fulfilled life.

We reveal the joy in experiencing the different generations, the love towards all that has been entrusted to us, and the sexual desire as deep inner volition towards the continuation of humankind.

Clear and consistent, we also protect and defend all this in readiness for an open confrontation.

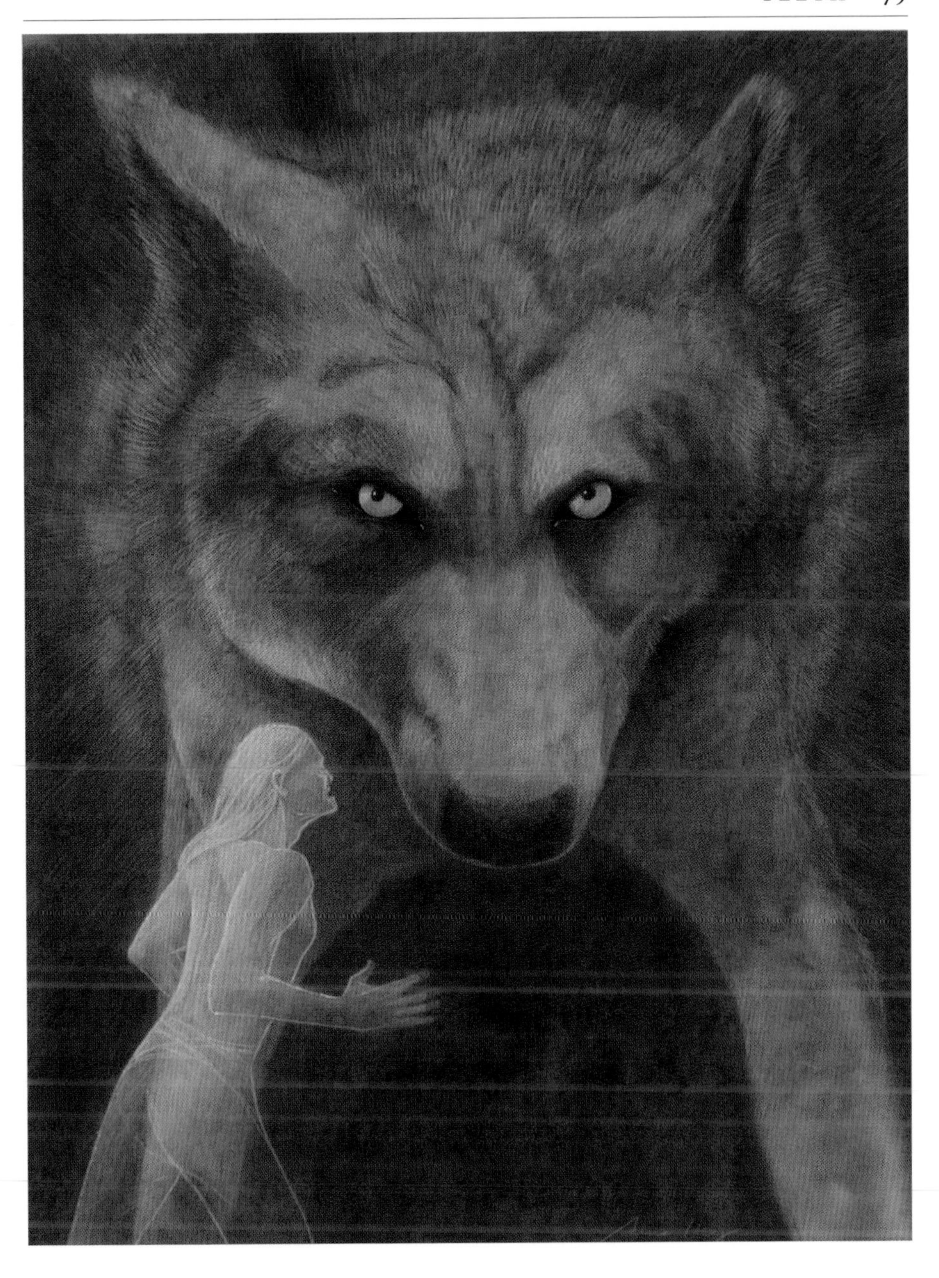

# Throat

To speak with the tongues of angels or sing like nightingales: In companionship with the breath my vocal cords bestow upon the human the expressiveness of words and the sound miracle of song.

My sounds are thereby as varied as the humans that generate them: Cooing, clicking, warbling, hissing, whistling or trilling; all this expresses thinking and, even more so, emotions.

After being formed the sounds receive their basic shapes and will then be fulfilled in the soundscapes of volume and depth. In that way, they reach people's hearts as tongue or voice, and on the inner level they fill all areas of body and soul.

Thus my structure is a mirror of the basic sentiments that bring understanding to both the inner and the outer.

"The mind is free!" – this topic is my concern and in deep love I loudly carry it outward so that it reaches the human being again in thousandfold reverberation. Moreover, as long as my posture is well tuned I can clearly sound my very own call to invite friends and lovers, but also use these elemental forces to defend against enemies and problems.

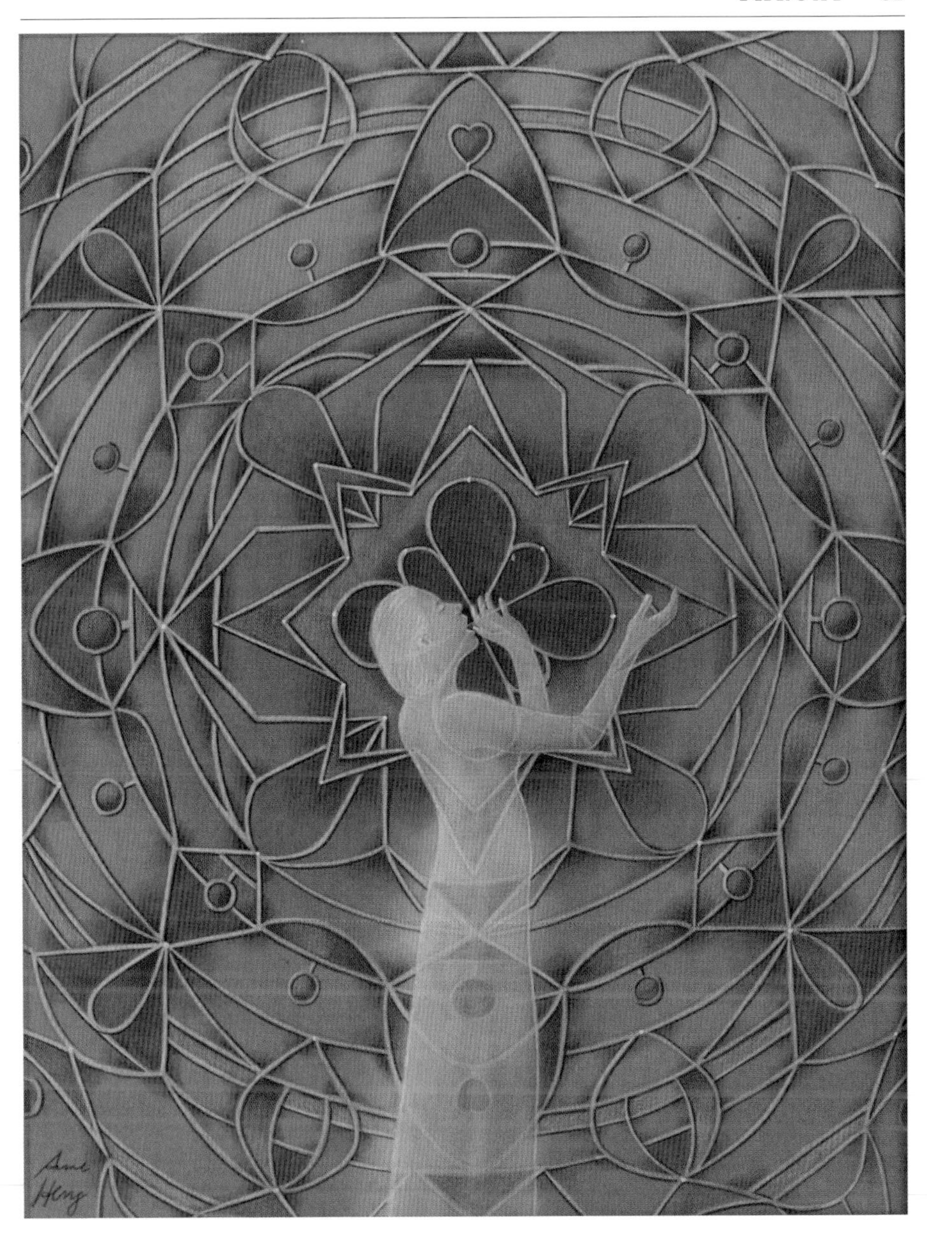

# Thymus

The Greeks of the ancient world gave me my name: "Thymos", the soul of breath, the breath of life.

Right they were, since from my place right underneath the breastbone I guard the energy portal of the heart and the inner energy currents. The themes I provide the human being with are called vitality and healthy self-determination.

I support the person through building a good immune system. With this, I defend body and soul against alien influences and protect every single human being in his or her very special uniqueness.

On the physical level it is predominantly viruses, bacteria and distorted cancer cells that threaten life, but I also protect the human on the soul level against damaging energies originating from stress, anger, envy or hatred.

My competence in solving problems allows me consistently, even in times of pressure, to conjure up a smile on people's faces; I exude trust from within my essence.

Thus I stabilize the protective shields that guard the energy layers of the aura. With the power of the "I am", the identity, originating from here, throughout life I provide the basis for health through fulfilment and honesty.

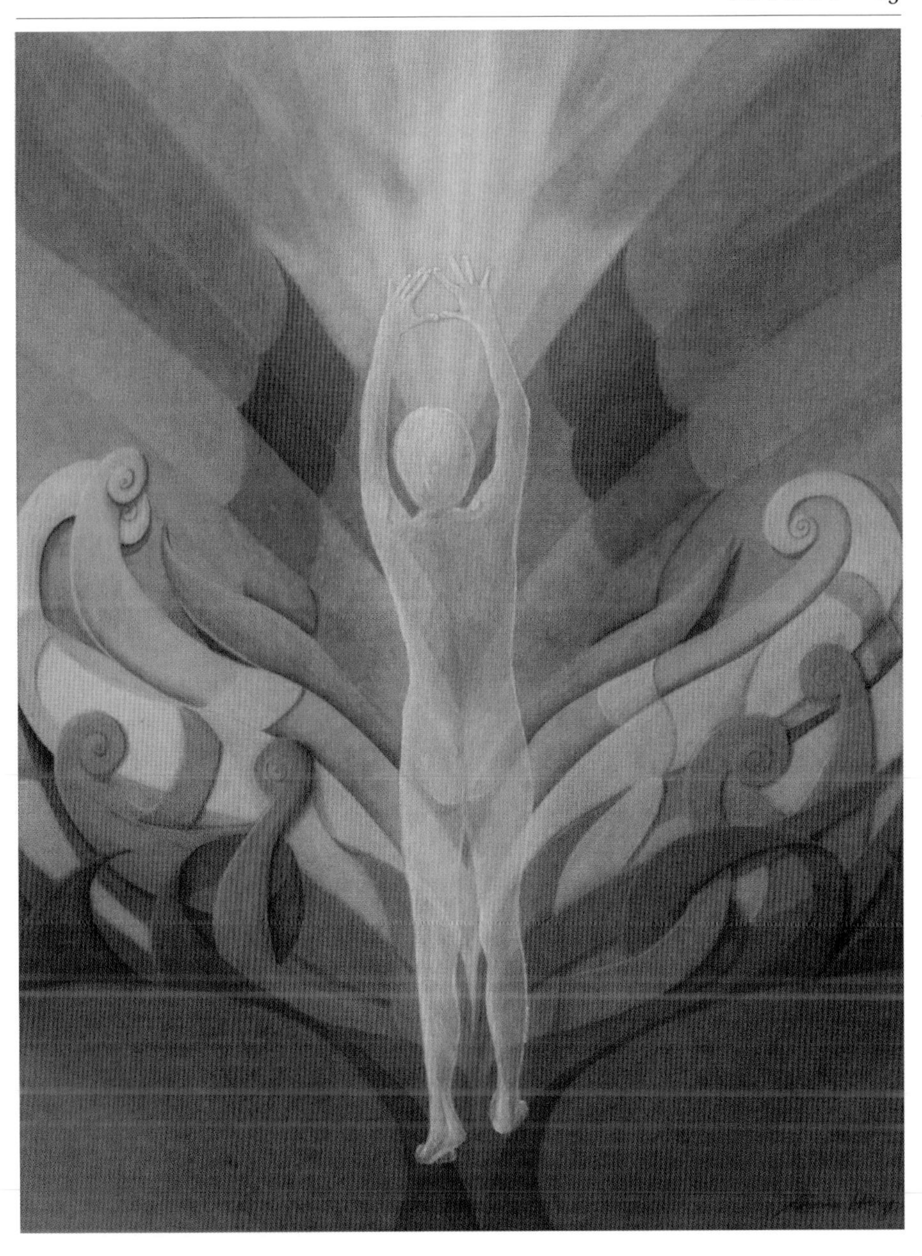

# Thyroid

When my hormone wings brush through the body's tissues with their gentle fire the cells are stimulated to higher activity. Through this, I support the transformation of food into energy and, further, into mental and soul potentials.

This metabolism ignites a true flight of sparks in body and soul, which activates the creativity, deepens the emotional stirrings and fuels the fire of sexuality. With the power of my firebird I carry the transformation in every experience.

In particular when the human being gets passionately involved in something, formations emerge that allow inner growth to occur and flourish step by step. This can develop into a burning, out of which ashes something new sprouts, which far exceeds the achieved.

If I am respected like this I can serve as firebird, sometimes ablaze or, equally, calmly enjoying that which has been achieved.
For this, I need a large and playful developmental space for the emotions and a loving understanding that keeps my fire under control. I feel at my best when thinking and feeling are in accord with the impulses of the inner fire.

Thereby people achieve a harmonious balance between a good basic tension and languorous letting go. This gives a guarantee of a fulfilled life.

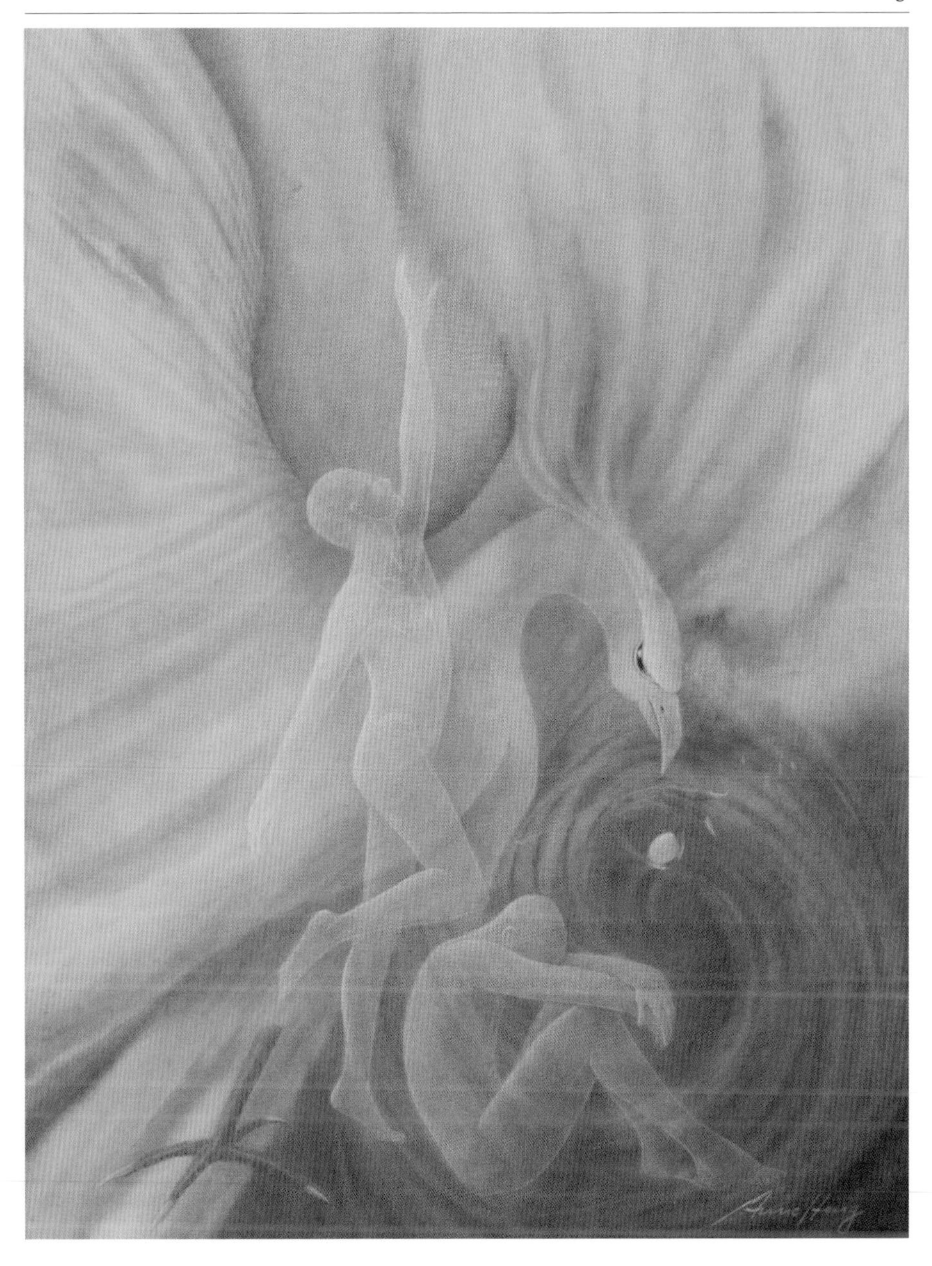

# Fundamentals

*The essence of things is hidden in the Unseen.*

*HERAKLIT*[11]

# Fundamentals – Stable but Intangible

As part of their understanding of life, all cultures describe an energetic field that lies beyond our physically tangible one. This has variously been denoted as "ether", "prana", "chi" and "breath". In this field the essence of the organs is present and awaits our attention.

Thus our contribution to this in this book was to call these pieces of information forward from the ether field and make them accessible in the form of written and painted illustrations. Through this process, we have been able to experience again and again how the elemental beings of the organs take effect.

When friends and clients tuned in to the paintings and texts they told us that they felt a tingling in their bodies; that waves of emotions flushed through them; that they were caught by spontaneous emotional reactions; that they had unusual dreams or that wonderful synchronicities happened. We also observed that within moments of tuning in changes took place: their facial features relaxed, their bodies straightened up and moved in a more aligned and fluid way, or their gaze became clearer and they spoke in a firmer voice. We gained more and more assurance in our assumption that the beings of the organs have a profound effect. Kinesiological tests confirmed these findings and thereby another piece of the puzzle fell into place.

*We know that outside of us exist neither colours nor sounds but exclusively vibrations. It is our brain that constructs a certain world out of this.*[12]

Traditional Chinese Medicine (TCM) identifies aspects of the organs that are connected with emotions, colours, sounds and even dreams.[13] Furthermore, they are linked with seasons and interwoven with the cosmic order. Here, at the frontiers of our imagination, the ether levels of the elemental beings begin; these elude rational thinking as their dimensions are too complex for us to grasp. Here, as mentioned before, the wisdom of timeless mystics corresponds with the evidence of modern atom physicists.

As passed on from Laozi (formerly known as Lao-tse) from the Daodejing (formerly titled Tao Te Ching): "The Dao one can speak of is not the eternal Dao."[14]

Equally paradoxical is this quote from Fritjof Capra: "There is movement though ultimately there are no moving objects; there is activity though no one who acts; there are no dancers but dance alone."[15]

We can also add here Hans-Peter Dürr:

> *At bottom there is no matter. At least not in the commonly used sense. There is only a network of relationships, constant change, aliveness. We find it difficult to imagine this. Primarily there is only correlation, the connecting without material basis. We could also call it spirit. Something that we can only experience spontaneously and not catch hold of. Matter and energy appear only secondarily – as coalgulated solidified spirit, in a manner of speaking.*[16]

# The Emergence of Reality

The fact that we cannot understand the whole of reality in its full dimension is connected to the way our brain works, as it is only in our brain that the world we call our reality is generated. Since the full reality of our world does not fit into our perception we select from the sum of the sense perceptions only those that we need for our survival. This adds up to only infinitesimal amounts of the total information[17] that reaches our sensory organs; the rest we reject. The remaining body of information we then amend and add it, in our brain, to our sentiments and thoughts to make up a whole picture that makes sense to us.

*The language is the clothing for our thoughts.*[18]

In this way we form a map of our reality. This construction of our reality is also the basis of language, which we use to convey our view of the world to others. We should, however, always be aware that with language we can only ever describe a map of reality.[19]

Thus it is easily comprehensible that the language of our linear mind is insufficient to describe the elemental beings, who live in the ether field beyond our imagination. If despite this we use language in order to make the essence of the organs available, we do so fully conscious of the fact that two people will read the same text in two different ways, and that there are as many ways to experience the world of the elemental beings as there are humans.

The same is, of course, true for the illustrations. Here too, every one of us will discover something different. As well as sensing our own organs' interior world and the individual interpretations of our perceptions, the elemental beings disclose two further gates through which we can reach them. One leads us through our intuition, or notions, and the other one presents itself to us through direct experience.

Notions and premonitions are very delicate and mostly not clear. We can neither grasp them nor relate them to anything. As unusual as this perspective appears, it is obvious that it is natural once we remember how we perceive the world. Looking at the two parts of the brain, it is the left part that predominantly provides our logical thinking, with the ability to gather details at an amazing speed. The right part of our brain is then responsible for assembling this wealth of individual information into a bigger whole. Here we can detect patterns and here we gain access to our notions and our intuition.

We all know situations in which we have seen something, and even if we were not able to say right away what it was, we had the feeling that we did in fact know it from somewhere. For our Neanderthal ancestors this was – in the worst-case scenario – a hungry cave bear; as best-case scenario the silhouettes of the returning hunters. The bear as well as the members of the tribe immediately evoked a wealth of emotions and thought connections, even before their appearance and identity became clear.

These kinds of perceptions we experience, in particular, unconsciously when dozing and consciously in deep meditation. We see or hear something ghostlike, blurred, without exactly knowing what it is. As soon as we activate the mind though we can identify this phenomenon as something that we know; then our brain substitutes the notion for something from our familiar conceptions. Thus a mystical experience transforms into the root of a tree, a waft of mist, an unusually sculpted group of plants or a collection of rock. If we keep the notion in suspense though, without activating the mind, it gains a meaning much bigger and more comprehensive than anything we can name.

Within the perception of notions we receive such an unbelievable concentration of information that we lack the words for it. Via the path of the notions we lend our senses to the organs' elemental beings and open ourselves up to their help. These are the moments where we experience ourselves as completely whole, or when out of a deep understanding we become aware of what it is that we need in order to become whole, and how we can have this turn into reality in our lives.

Usually, this condition is connected with a deep experience of happiness. Words fail us during a direct experience of the organs' elemental beings. Such moments are so charged that our thinking comes to a stop. At such a moment, an inconceivable cornucopia of information pours out into our awareness and we share in the wonder of an organ. Then we suddenly and abruptly find ourselves within a cell that reveals how it operates in its profound tunings. We become aware of the cell's molecular and atomic structures, simultaneously experience the history it carries, and receive pictures from an indescribable timelessness of being.

These are the moments in which we are directly connected with existence, where we are the cell as well as the observer and where we know that the universe is whole. From this point onwards everything will be different, even if it seemingly, on the surface, continues in the same way.

*Symbols bring out our original nature.*[20]

# Our Channels for the Organ Beings

In notions and premonitions, as well as in those moments when we directly experience the elemental beings of the organs, we need different channels. These include pictures, words and sounds that touch us in our soul. Our soul processes a multitude of information as the pure picture that we see or the sole sound that we hear.

"The bluish gleam of a thin china cup brings back childhood memories. I know that I can take the cup and pour tea into it. If it falls onto the floor it will break." This example, from Christof Koch,[21] illustrates the importance of symbols in daily life. But symbols go much further than this.

Carl Gustav Jung described them, in his writings on the archetypes, as figures within the human soul that exist in all peoples. They point towards basic soul principles that operate within us. Examples for this are the fairy godmother, the evil witch, the hero or the inner child.

Moore and Gillette have likened the operating mechanism of archetypes quite explicitly to iron filings spread on a piece of paper underneath which a magnet is moved around.[22] The movement of the iron filings that is visible to us corresponds to our perceptible soul movements, while the magnet is the operating of our archetypal inner soul forces, which direct our personality from the shadows.

In symbols reality is condensed into the most essential. Thus we can recognize ourselves in them as in a mirror and make peace with our nature. To do this we fill the symbol in our consciousness with life, with content from our past, with fantasies and with sensations/sentiments from all levels of being. Thereby we add to the symbol until it takes on an inner presence of its own.

The depictions of the organs' essences are symbolic forms of poetry that we collect from the ether field. The most important aspect here lies in what we read between the lines and what we see hiding behind the picture. Often we cannot grasp this immediately and sometimes it is even irritating, since different time and space dimensions flow together here towards one point of perception.

If, however, we open ourselves up to this, synchronicities and insights all assemble into a whole that makes sense and leads to a deeper connection with life, and ultimately to a comprehensive experience of "being whole". When we thus engage with the organ beings we experience our body as a wonderful concert in which the organs create with highest virtuosity the sound miracle of our body. This is the symphony that carries us through life.

> *Never having heard the voice of God and his angels is considered a sign of health by the world.*[23]

# We Are An Idea of the Soul

All this becomes possible through the nature of the organ's elemental beings, who as original soul ideas of the organs are at home within the backdrop of existence, where the information and energies of life flow. Through them we thus gain a different appreciation of our body and experience a better unison of body and soul, which just renders unsuitable ways of life no longer necessary.

It is even more essential here to move beyond habitual thought patterns and view our existence from a higher perspective. As human beings we are first and foremost an idea of the soul, a soul field that fills itself with energies, matter and functions according to the individual requirements and characteristics of our life plan.

Or expressed differently: The soul has created a body from the divine essence of our being, so that we can have experiences on earth in this human form. The organs are hereby the pillars of the life functions that guarantee that we exist at all on our planet.

It is not only the biochemical processes of the body that are part of this. Equally important for our survival are the organs' functional complexes. Thus the kidneys are not only in charge of the body's harmonious water balance but also of the soul's balance in the areas of perseverance, willpower and confidence; and as

When we thus engage with the organ beings we experience our body as a wonderful concert in which the organs create with highest virtuosity the sound miracle of our body.

well as digestion the stomach takes care of equanimity in the areas of conflict management as well as of the inner fire that transforms desires into insights.

This connection becomes very obvious in the example of the spleen. In conventional medicine, the spleen is only considered when it needs to be removed, while in Traditional Chinese Medicine (TCM) as well as in Traditional European Naturopathy (TEN) it is awarded extremely significant energetic functions. In TCM the energy of the spleen is responsible for storage and distribution of the flowing energies, for preservation of the building energy and for the ability to think, to ponder and to sing.

Within TEN, our ancestors equally recognized the energetic tasks of the spleen and credited it with the ability to remove stressful energies during the transformational processes of our food in our bodies. Thus the spleen also throws the gloom out of the (spiritual) home. In TEN this depressing mental–emotional condition is connected with the concepts of "black bile" and "melancholia".

Through such energetic actions our organs act as physical compensation fields so that we can intercept excessive demands on the soul and process them well. In order to cope better with stress, for example, we increase our muscle tone. Our posture changes when we are happy or when we are sad and when we cannot cope with soul conflicts our organs make themselves known with physical discomfort. This is the potential for compensating that we know of from psychosomatic medicine.

Equally, very sensitive people sense conflicts in their environment in the form of physical discomfort or pain. Often they are even able to solve the problem through inner processing of these conflicts.

We also know of this phenomenon from shamans of diverse cultures past and present. To heal their patients' illnesses they go on an inner shamanic journey and resolve the issues in question on the spiritual level. That we are all interwoven in an incredible network of spiritual connections should be obvious just from looking at the example of clinical psychologist Dr. Hew Len in a Hawaii prison hospital: He was applying deep Hawaiian Ho'oponopono healing work to himself and through this healed a whole ward full of people. He achieved this through simply studying the files of mentally ill high-risk offenders. It should be added here that Dr. Len had never personally met a single one of these inmates.[24]

> *A rose is a rose only because the human perceives it as such; without the human it would only be a pattern of energy vortices.*[25]

# How Real is Our Reality?

In order to get along in our world we have, thanks to our faculty of speech, coined abstract concepts. Hereby we have named things. Proceeding from there we have also conceptually named our activities. If we think about this carefully, we can see that we have thus "frozen" processes and thereby transformed something that is by nature continuously flowing into a static "thing".

Thus, for example, something that we explain has become an "explanation"; the way we ride a bus, a "ride", or what we think, a "thought". However, in contrast to planks, stones, tables or chairs that we can touch, explanations, rides and thoughts are intangible. This also applies to conditions of being like joy, happiness or grief, which we can indeed experience but which are also intangible.

Unfortunately, we have drawn the bow even tauter and also classified "life", "love", our "self" or even our "soul" or "God" as something tangible, without recognising the fact that we only experience all this in ways that are beyond our thinking and, in fact, completely elude access or understanding through our mind.[26]

Quantum physics has added a further dimension since we had to recognize that classical mechanical physics reaches its limits where anything living is concerned.

But we can touch our bodies! Yes, and on a certain level they are very tangible. But if we look more closely we are confronted with the mystery of life. The neurosciences can still not tell us how and where we store our memories.[27]

Possibly our brain functions as a great processor that uses an information repository in the ether field.[28] Science actually assumes that we construct our memories anew every moment,[29] and even for such seemingly clear functions like those of our cells we ultimately have mere explanatory models that are continuously replaced by new insights.

All these almost unsolvable mysteries are illuminated when we consider ourselves as consciousness. Then we can understand that the organs' elemental beings represent collective consciousness from the etheric field, which is at our disposal to create the forms and functions of the organs.

Medical progress has encouraged us to consider the body as an object, so it is not surprising that our language when it comes to organs no longer has anything much to do with us as spiritual beings. Our medical language has truly become soulless, and not just because of all the Latin and Greek expressions. Accordingly, our medical professionals work at the level of having to repair "faulty" organs, or sometimes even exchange them.

Traditional healing modalities view all of this rather differently. They consider illness to be an expression of an imbalance of psychological, energetic and physical processes. They understand that it is not only the symptoms that need to be treated but also the underlying mental and spiritual issues. Otherwise the problems will simply re-emerge in a different form and at a different place.

Thus the path of natural healing modalities consists in supporting the person concerned to rediscover their own inner balance. Our conventional medicine, on the other hand, sees enemies everywhere: bacteria, viruses, harmful pollen or a sinister environment that needs fighting.

At times it is not even very clear who or what the battles are actually directed at; and with this approach, very often it is the very body that we are trying to heal that loses out. With all respect to modern medicine: Life works differently. Thus Gadamer[30] was right when he said that the body is measurable in its functions, but the frame is fitted.

At this point in human history, when we have veered drastically into thinking like machines, the spiritual levels of life are coming forward again. In their essence portraits the elemental beings reflect the perfect harmony of our organs and ourselves. Hereby each of these organ beings presents itself in its core statement with the message: "I am a part of you with my organ!"

Through our awareness the organ beings bring attention to these basic features of spirit in our bodies and indicate how we can fulfil our potential in life through our own very personal form of expression. To this effect, elemental beings with their organs are gifts of life itself, and help us to rediscover harmony in our body and become whole.

Even when an organ needs to be removed, the corresponding elemental being is by no means without a home in the person's body. The form of an organ always follows a function, which themselves follow an idea.

In their essence portraits the elemental beings reflect the perfect harmony of our organs and ourselves.

This can be observed very well in the interplay of muscles and bones: When a muscle is being trained through exercise it anchors itself more strongly in the bone, which grows firmer at that particular point in order to provide the muscle with a better hold.

Our health is heavily based on such compensatory abilities, where bones can compact, where areas of the brain can take on different functions after a stroke, or where after a spleen removal the liver can move in to take on most of the spleen's tasks. These compensations happen thanks to the organ beings, who first and foremost are an integral part of ideas and functions, and only in a secondary way part of their physical organ tissue.

Ultimately, the organ beings organize our survival – from integrating into other systems to organizing the whole body anew and to organs growing again after being removed.

*Complete healing and spiritual awakening are really one and the same.*[31]

# The Recurrent Theme of Healing

If we speak of getting closer to the organs' elemental beings, this is not quite correct as, through the very fact of our lives, we are already inseparably connected with them. Thus ultimately we need to remember that the energy and information currents of our spiritual soul consciousness comprise the body as well, and that we are a unity of soul and body.

This knowledge is always available to us. Whether we are working, eating, loving or sleeping, it is our awareness alone that opens us up to the power of the elemental beings.

Wise ones, healers and shamans have over centuries provided pathways for us in order to facilitate access to this consciousness. There is a recurrent theme in healing that runs through all cultures and methods. It does not matter if we are dealing with open heart surgery, a naturopathic herb prescription or a reiki session.

There are three components that open the pathways for our personal spiritual growth and in which we find the foundation of all healing treatments.[32]

- At our spiritual/inner place of silence, where the unconscious chatter of the mind is silent, we can listen to our inner voice without bias. Through this, we receive essential impulses that inform our actions.
- In this body we have the chance of experiencing our inner purpose. This includes a Yes to life and the willingness to fulfil our tasks therein with enthusiasm.

- In our uniqueness we are part of the universe that would not be whole without us. This mystery of life beyond our mind we can only experience through love and dedication.

*Life is not a problem that we need to solve, but a reality that wants to be experienced.*[33]

# We Arrive at a Place of Inner Tranquility

Even when we just gaze at the organ beings in their portraits in a relaxed way we experience a pause in the habitual flow of our thinking, and our perception opens up to the deeper levels of our being. With this we can access, through our notions, the opportunity to hear our inner voice more clearly. In which form we are then going to realize these indications is another question.

Even if we do not implement what we have received immediately, this inner listening gives us more peace. Our soul is timeless, which is why it has infinitely more patience than our mind. Just through gazing and opening up to notions a gap arises in our "inner chatter". Thus an inner place of silence opens, in which we receive the most important information for our life.

This is a space that we can call on during a meditation; it can open up for us in the hustle and bustle of a farmers' market and we can experience it in the transitions between sleeping and waking. It can be accessible to us for days and weeks, or a blink of an eye can suffice to learn the most essential knowledge from our inner being.

This might suggest to us a topic that changes the course of a meeting, it can influence decisions in our relationship with our partner, and it can concern the composition of our shopping list in the supermarket. Some people let their thoughts wander to a place that they know from their childhood, others find the gateway to their inner space in the spaciousness of the blue sky or in the tip of the pencil they are holding.

Once that place is reached, the outer world seems to fade into the background. In this time, we experience a stillness, where reality becomes incredibly clearly perceptible and where at the same time we receive our inner voice unbiased. Thus the organ beings bring us into a presence in the Here and Now where we are in touch with the essence of life.

At the same time this reconnection makes the attunements between soul, personality and body more permeable. Even though the inner voice of the elemental beings can be quite inconvenient as it can bring up things that we find difficult, it still always reflects back to us those aspects of our lives that move us forward on a soul level. Thereby it becomes easier to shift obstacles and to let our joie de vivre grow. Ultimately this paves the way to health and healing.

> *Existence is delicious – we only need to have the courage to lead our own life.*[34]

# A Decision for Life

To live our own creativity in a self-determined way – this may be one of the most difficult tasks there is. Although we should first dispel a misconception – this does not mean that we just "do our thing" without regard for others. It is better thought of as a service of love for our community in attunement with ourselves. This involves a benevolent intention and loving mindfulness, towards ourselves as well as others.

If something unfair or hostile to life is happening, though, firm and clear words are needed and they may not necessarily be well received by everyone. Nevertheless, the keys to a wholesome self-determination in life remain the same: Love, truthfulness and connection. In this way of living, we are increasingly called to give more space to a Yes to life. It is a form of love in which we expand above the familiar and employing the three keys mentioned helps us to embrace the mystery of life.

We can truly see the happiness in people who live such an inner connection. This inner connection also very positively affects our spiritual and physical health. When we are in tune with ourselves our movements become more fluent, the inner processes of our body chemistry can work better and our awareness also gains clarity. These are examples of having a good presence in our bodies, and it is this that the organs' elemental beings support us with. Moreover, they help

To live our own creativity in a self-determined way – this may be one of the most difficult tasks there is.

us with handling crises, convey wholesome impulses with regard to illnesses that threaten us and reflect back on us their perfect love in our being. Above all, though, they show us that life carries us and that day-to-day concerns such as our performance in our profession or in other areas are not the most important things. More, the organs' elementals invite us to celebrate the whole of our existence with active participation and enthusiasm. Thus we can fulfill our life task with creativity and full of joy.

> *Fifty years of intense pondering have brought me no closer to the answer to the question: "What are light quanta?"*[35]

# We Are Unique – Even If We Do Not Understand It

When we grapple with life, sooner or later we touch the basic levels of our being. These levels cannot be grasped with the mind; we can experience them only in their mysteries. Through reflecting on the spiritual roots of our existence, healers and sages have always realized that we are part of the divine and that the universe will only be whole through our own very personal contribution.

We do, however, seem to reach our limits when trying to understand human nature. Thus Max Planck concluded, approaching this question through quantum physics: "Science cannot solve the last riddles of nature. It cannot achieve this because we are a part of nature ourselves and thus also a part of the riddle that we want to solve."[36]

Max Planck and a long line of physicists shook up our view of the world when they started considering the nature of matter in a new light. For so long matter had been assumed to be firm and stable, but these scientists discovered that we have to view matter as aggregations of frequency fields. We can still shatter a windowpane by throwing a stone through it; however, at the level of the atomic particles, stone as well as windowpane as well as the person who has hurled the stone consist – to an incredibly large percentage – of empty space in which energies circle.

And if we look at that one-billionth of seemingly solid matter, the atom nucleus, what remains ultimately is only energy potentials, frequencies and resonances, an insight for which Carlo Rubbia received the Nobel Prize in 1984.

But this truth was described 5,000 years ago by ancient Indian wise ones with the concept and phrase "nada brahma": "The world is sound." This ancient tenet of Indian spirituality conveys the meaning and the knowledge that everything in the universe is based on vibrations, that the world is effectively a huge concert, in which we are all an instrument: a symphony in which the great consciousness, the all One, plays itself.

> *Consciousness is empty in its nature. And it still comprises and holds all things.*[37]

Since the beginning of the twentieth century, frequencies and resonances have made for a scientific revolution in biology as well as physics. Research in molecular biology had up to that point predominantly focused on the substances, the so-called facts, but in the Seventies the study of biophotons opened a new chapter in the study of the science of life.[38]

Through this pioneering research, we can now illuminate the inner calibration of our life functions and it becomes obvious that the organs are not simply cell aggregates that function more or less randomly. Rather, they are highly organized structures in which the cells communicate via a laser-like light in an electromagnetic field. This communication via light is one of the bridges to consciousness.

It was physicists who concluded from investigating subatomic particles that we have to concede a form of consciousness to even the tiniest structures of matter. With this insight we may finally understand the universe as an enormous field of consciousness into which we are integrated.

Then of course every organ has a presence in this field; moreover, an organ is a consciousness that is linked with everything.

Neuroscience has a different understanding of consciousness than depth psychology, and quantum physics has a completely different conception again.

According to the insights of quantum physics, the two electrons that make up the hydrogen atom, the simplest atom in existence, know of each other. A good friend and biophysicist provided a lovely explanation for this during a diverting car journey: When a group of soldiers marches and has for some reason to scatter left and right into the bushes, the individual members are still aware of each other and still perceive themselves as a unity, despite the physical dispersal.

This form of consciousness continues beyond atoms: Beyond molecules, cell systems, organs and humans, right up to us living all together on our planet – and even beyond that we are integrated into the whole universe.

> *Unpredictability distinguishes the animate being from robots. It is what makes life unique and peculiar, even though occasionally also difficult.*[39]

# Organs Are Condensed Consciousness of Love

Professor Popp can provide conclusive evidence that the perfect performances of animate beings are made possible by the electromagnetic frequency fields of the biophotons. Hereby every atom and every cell is drawn into an exact position in a holographic field and anchored there. These precise calibrations in our organism are possible through intelligent fields within us of biophotons of the highest order.

Only a consciousness, i.e. a cognitive awareness of oneself, can maintain the regulations of life functions in which about ten million body cells are substituted each second. Interesting as well that each organ knows exactly when it has enough cells and which overall form as organ these cells are supposed to build. But how does the organ know that? An answer to these questions of life is still owed us by conventional medical science.

We are at the deepest level connected with everything. We can see this just by looking at our blood and other bodily fluids; they are composed of minerals and trace elements in the same ratio as the seawater in our oceans.[40] We can equally clearly read our affiliation to the universe in the vibrations through which we are woven into the biological system of our earth: Our body shows a basic resonance of 7–13 hertz. The same frequency, the so-called Schumann resonance, can be found in our brainwaves when we are relaxed. The crust as well as the ionosphere of our earth pulsate in this same frequency.[41]

Thus we can see that we are in an optimal interaction with the consciousness field of the earth; and with the whole of existence. From the orbits of the two electrons in the hydrogen[42]atom to the human being the calibrations became more and more complex and expansive. Each evolutionary step has been able to combine within itself more comprehensive and more complex conditions, as F. A. Popp demonstrated.[43] At this point current science re-connects with the paradoxes of the mystics of the past, who said that the world is perfect at all times and that at the same time it is always striving towards even greater perfection.

If we go further and search for the roots of the matter, we discover sooner or later that the whole of existence is based not on matter but on a spiritual principle. This is true for the windowpane as much as for the stone and also for our "I am" or our identity, as well as for our body with its organs and cells. This spiritual principle connects everything in its creative force, and goes beyond cells, molecules, electromagnetic fields and even space and time. It is a form of intelligence that lives within us, a consciousness of love.

Out of this source the elemental beings of the organs are energized too. They ensure that the universal vibrations in our body can construct themselves into organs with their manifold physical and spiritual functions. Seen in this way, our organs are condensed love.

> *The first drink from the cup of science creates atheists; but at the bottom of the cup God is waiting.*[44]

The topic of organs and their elemental beings inevitably touches again and again on different modes of healing. In order to prevent misunderstandings: Even when we engage with the organs in this form we will not be spared the occasional experience of illness. Through our "willing participation in the maelstrom of life"[45] we sometimes need pointers and support in recovering our inner wisdom.

The difference from conventional medicine's way of handling illness, though, lies in lovingly connecting with the organs and their elemental beings, and asking them what they need in order to rediscover their optimal calibration with the consciousness fields of body and universe. Healing is hereby not at all a passive process or restricted to one human level. It is a path on which we support our body mentally–spiritually, energetically, naturopathically and also with conventional medicine. Linked to this are a turning towards the inner and an opening up to the loving intelligence of our body.

In this way the organs' beings can unfold their magnificent capacities, without being burdened by the contradictions of the mind and detached from the constraints that we have imposed upon ourselves. Inviting the organs' elemental beings into our life in this way does not make medicine redundant; it simply makes it more humane and awards a new dignity to everyone involved.

> *Everything I say, be talk, nothing be an advice. I would not speak as boldly if one had to follow me.*[46]

# Notes

1 Christian Morgenstern (1871–1914)
2 Gadamer, Hans-Georg (1900–2002), *The Enigma of Health: The Art of Healing in a Scientific Age*. Palo Alto, CA: Stanford University Press, 1996.
3 Dürckheim, Karlfried Graf (1896–1988), *Vom doppelten Ursprung des Menschen*. Rütte: Johanna Nordländer Verlag, 2009.
4 Angelus Selesius (1624–1677), *The Cherubinic Wanderer*. Heaven is within you. Maria Shrady (ed.). Mahwah, NJ: Paulist Press, 1986.
5 Archetypes are described within part 3, *Fundamentals*, at the end of the book.
6 Catharina Regina von Greiffenberg (1633–1694)
7 Teresa of Avila (1515–1582)
8 Kliegel, E., *Reflexzonen – Landkarten der Gesundheit*. CD-ROM, 2009.
9 Hildegard von Bingen (1098–1179) *Physika* – from Gienger, M., *Die Heilsteine der Hildegard von Bingen*. Saarbrücken: Neue Erde, 2004.
10 Gienger et al., *Crystal Massage for Health and Healing*. Forres: Earthdancer/Findhorn Press, 2006.
11 Heraklit (ca. 520–460 B.C.)
12 Jäger, Willigis, *Die Welle ist das Meer, Mystische Spiritualität*. 24th edition. Freiburg: Herder, 2011.
13 This Chinese standard medical work is attributed to the legendary Yellow Emperor Huang-ti who is said to have lived in 2,700 B.C. The Nei Ching was written in the times of the Warring States Period (221 B.C.–220 A.C.).
14 The Daodejing (mostly known as Tao Te Ching) is attributed to the legendary Laozi (Old Master) and originates in the 6th century BC.
15 Capra, F., *The Turning Point: Science, Society, and the Rising Culture*. New York: Bantam Books, 1983/1988.
16 Dürr, H.-P., "Am Anfang war der Quantengeist", interview in *P.M. Magazin* (Mai 2007).

17 Hubel, D. H., "Auge und Gehirn, Neurobiologie des Sehens", *Spektrum*, Heidelberg, 1988.
18 Samuel Johnson (1709–1784)
19 Based on Alfred Korzybski (1879–1950).
20 Jung, C. G. (1875–1961), *Man and his symbols.* F. P. C. Verlag 1964.
21 Koch, C., *Bewußtsein–ein neurologisches Rätsel.* Elsevier, München, 2005.
22 Moore, R. / Gillette, D., *King, Warrior, Magician, Lover: Rediscovering the Archetypes of the Mature Masculine.* New York: Harper Collins, 1991.
23 Sri Aurobindo (1872–1950)
24 Starkmuth, J., *Fragen und Antworten zur Realität*, supplementary volume to *The Making of Reality.* Bonn: Starkmuth Publishing, 2011.
25 E. H. Shattuk, quoted from Starkmuth, ibid.
26 Starkmuth, J., *The Making of Reality.* 10th edition. Bonn: Starkmuth Publishing, 2009.
27 Starkmuth, J., ibid.
28 Bischof, M., *Biophotonen, Das Licht in unseren Zellen.* Frankfurt/M.: Zweitausendeins, 1995.
29 Kortre, J., *White Gloves: How We Create Ourselves Through Memory.* New York: W. W. Norton & Company Inc., 1996.
30 Gadamer, H.-G., *The Enigma of Health: The Art of Healing in a Scientific Age.*
31 Tarthang Tulku (Tibetan Lama)
32 This listing originates in its basic structure from: Carlson, R., Shield, B., *Healers on Healing*, in particular: Richard Moss and Shakti Gawain. New York: Jeremy P. Tarcher, 1992.
33 Buddha (Siddhartha Gautama ca. 563–483 BC)
34 Peter Rosegger (1843–1918)
35 Albert Einstein (1879–1955)
36 Max Planck (1858–1947)
37 Tilopa (988–1069) – *The Ganges Mahamudra*
38 Popp, F. A., *Biophotonen–neue Horizonte in der Medizin: von den Grundlagen zur Biophotonik.* Stuttgart: MVS, 2006.
39 Popp, F. A., *Die Botschaft der Nahrung. Unsere Lebensmittel in neuer Sicht.* Frankfurt/M.: Zweitausendeins, 2011.
40 Lipton, H. B., *Biology of Belief: Unleashing the Power of Consciousness, Matter & Miracles.* Revised edition. Carlsbad, CA: Hay House, 2011.
41 Bischof, M., *Biophotonen, Das Licht in unseren Zellen.*
42 Hydrogen is nearly always found as H2 double atom.
43 Popp, F. A., *Biophotonen–neue Horizonte in der Medizin: von den Grundlagen zur Biophotonik.*
44 Paracelsus (1493–1541)
45 Osborn, M. / Longland, S., *Rune Games.* London: Penguin Books, 1988.
46 Erasmus of Rotterdam (1465–1536)

And a special thanks to the stunning researches of Lynne McTaggart in her book *The Field: The Quest for the Secret Force of the Universe.* London: Element/HarperCollins, 2003.

# About the Authors

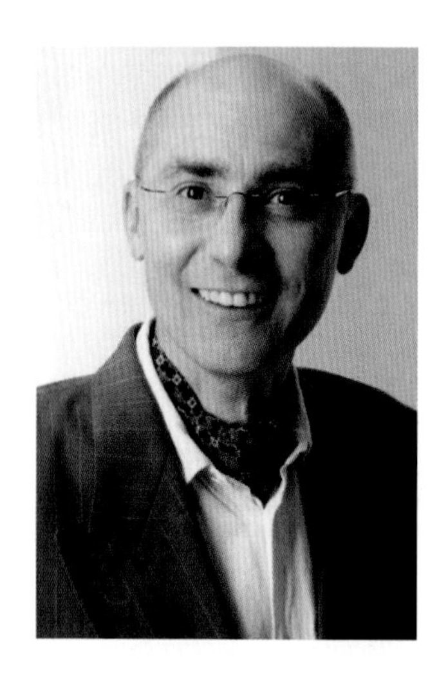

EWALD KLIEGEL (born 1957)
Ewald's professional engagement with people began with two work placements in 1976: One took him to a urological hospital, the other one to a school for children with learning disabilities. Since then, healing and teaching alike have formed a thread throughout his life. His medical trainings as a massage therapist and naturopath have paved the way to his holistic perspective on body and soul. Since 1989, he has taught at naturopathy schools as well as in his own seminars in Germany and abroad.

With his maps Reflexzonen: Landkarten der Gesundheit (Reflexology: Maps of Health), published in 1992, he found a consistent formal vocabulary for depicting more than thirty reflexology systems. In 1996, crystal wands were added to his work as energy tools that he developed for reflexology and acupressure treatments. Around 1999, Ewald started his research for the book Reflexzonen und Organsprache (Reflexology and the Language of the Organs), which was published in 2008. Here the organs were no longer portrayed as a medium of illnesses; instead, they were expressed, in diverting stories, as archetypal pictures of the soul that affect our most inner being. Continuing from here, Ewald follows the organs into the spiritual metaphysical fundamentals of our being where they show themselves in the light of their own essence and idea of creation. This has been illustrated magnificently by Anne Heng.

In seminars of his programme "Reflex–Balance", Ewald Kliegel teaches reflexology and crystal treatments for therapy and professional wellness. He also offers presentations, events and seminars in which he opens up space for the psychological and soul aspects of the organs, where self-awareness, mindfulness and meditative approach help construct a healing field for a deeper connection with the organs. These events lend themselves to improving body awareness as well as serving as mind and soul healthcare.

Contact:

Ewald Kliegel
Rotenbergstr. 154
70190 Stuttgart
Germany
info@reflex-balance.eu
www.reflex-balance.eu

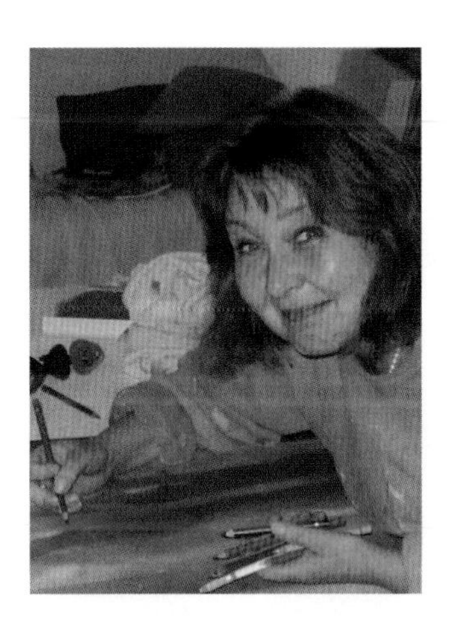

ANNE HENG (born 1953)
Anne has studied art and design and joyfully spends her time as a painter, illustrator and awareness teacher. Her special technique of painting on silk enables her to harmoniously interweave flowing and concrete aspects, dream and reality, intuition and skill. Since 1986, she has worked as a freelance artist with many exhibitions in Germany and abroad, and as an illustrator for various publishers.

It is her wish to touch people's hearts with her work and to open them to the unobtrusive quiet beauty of nature. Anne lives with her husband, her son and several cats in an old schoolhouse in Weilburg, Germany.

In her contribution to Ewald Kliegel's idea and vision, Anne has painted the organs as strong symbols with an intense and unique vibrancy. The pictures show the personalities of the organs and speak through their love, gentleness and strength directly to the soul; more, they offer a reconnection with the essence of the organs and facilitate access to what happens in your own body.

*Drawing is my meditation,*
*the exploration of spiritual worlds my passion.*
*If both comes together it feels like pure joy.*

Contact:

Anne Heng
Schulbergstr. 9
35781 Weilburg
Germany
MiAnHeng@aol.com
www.anne-heng.de



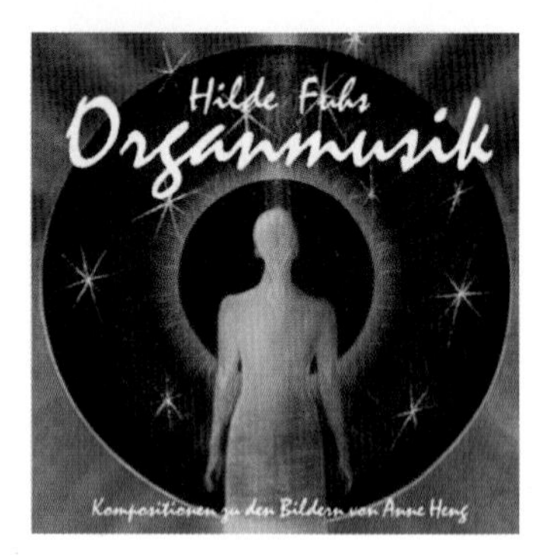